BLACK BELT YOGA

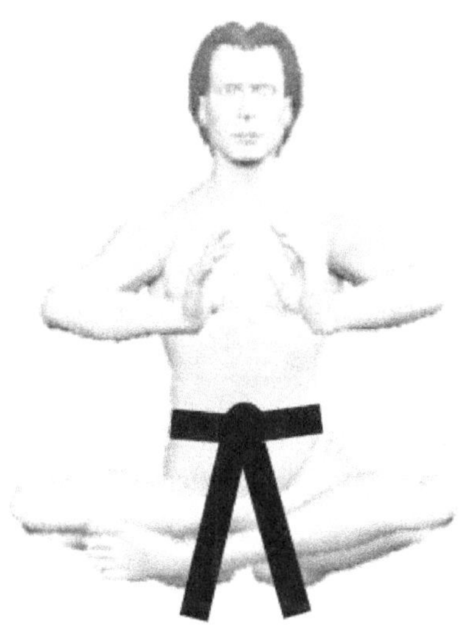

AL CASE

QUALITY PRESS

Copyright © 2024 by Alton H. Case

The author may be reached through

MonsterMartialArts.com,

AlCaseBooks.com

obligatory warning

The US government has deemed that it is against the law to cure anybody, and they are so-o-o right. You're going to have to do it yourself. So use the things in this tome, and if you don't end up curing yourself, keep looking and keep working and dedicate yourself to good health. Boy, that'll really piss the government off. Heh.

introduction

Yoga, and a Black Belt. Hmmm.

Well, martial arts are a structure of motion, and they lead to enlightenment.

Yoga is non-motion, and it leads to enlightenment.

Do you see the similarities of the two?

So why not use the structure of the martial arts, with its belt ranking system, to better order Yoga, and to insure that people more easily progress to enlightenment?

The above said, let me describe what you will encounter on this path.

There are four disciplines, those of the monk, the yogi, the warrior (Martial Artist), and ascetic.

Each discipline has elements necessary to enlightenment.

It is my purpose to blend those elements and to define the whole picture of enlightenment.

It is my purpose to blend those disciplines so that one travels faster and more surely to enlightenment.

The truth of the matter is that the enlightenment to be gained is the same for each discipline. We travel in the same universe, we fight the same elements, but we give the individual battles different names, describe phenomena from different points of view.

But if you understand each of those points of view, you will better understand the whole picture, and you will travel faster and more surely to enlightenment.

I will be using something called Neutronics to make the four disciplines mesh.

Neutronics is based on the 'unmoving' part of the atom. Neutronics is a study of the only thing in this universe that can't be measured...Awareness. That means that Neutronics is the science of...you.

Behind the eyes and ears, behind the muscles and neurons, behind every motion in this universe, is a human being, an 'I am,' a...you.

So we take apart and blend the four disciplines so that you will see what they are and how they can fit together.

We make a path, a larger path, a true Fourfold Path, that will be faster and more sure, and lead to...you.

And, my apologies, you are going to find certain ragged edges in this tome. This is because what I am doing, what I am presenting here, has never before been presented.

This is the true Fourfold Path, and it has never been seen in the affairs of man.

That's okay. We're going to have fun, anyway.

WHITE BELT

There have been ranking systems in every institution ever since there were two people. Adam presided over Eve, every Indian has his Chief, and so on.

And, in every army there has been a chain of command which consists of levels (private, sergeant, etc.) So rank isn't a new thing. And, in the west we usually break things down to beginner, intermediate, advanced, and so on.

The martial arts breakdown of belt levels is somewhat more unique. You see, more is happening in the martial arts. People are are not learning more easily learned knowledge, such as math or science or whatever. They are learning the more difficult to measure experience of awareness.

The first martial arts belt system was probably introduced in swimming classes in Okinawa or Japan, but the martial arts glommed on to that thing real quick.

I'm a higher belt so I am tougher. That's a selling point if ever there was one.

But, in Yoga, we have two things to consider.

One, a person's ability in holding (controlling) a body posture.

Two, the level of awareness required to hold such a posture.

That said, you may zoom through the first few belt levels, possibly in a day. But then the going gets tougher, and you now have to sit in posture, and you may not have the discipline that doing the easy poses generates.

You may need to take the time to stretch and make flexible the body.

So even if you can zoom through, don't.

Take a few hours, make the ability to sit, and ponder, and do actual meditation, grow. (In the next discourse you will find exact definitions of Meditation, so there will be no confusion on that point).

Remember, it's not just the ability to make the body hold posture, it is the awareness generated by that ability. These two things, discipline (of posture) and awareness go hand in glove, and it is advised that you do not take your hand out of the glove until you have thoroughly examined each posture, and gleaned from them the rudimentary beginnings of becoming a disciplined, aware, human being.

MEDITATION

Ask somebody what meditation is and they'll frequently give you a mysterious look, and say some odd thing that titillates like, 'That is the question, isn't it?'

Well, I don't expect you to get somewhere without a roadmap, so let's define meditation succinctly and exactly and forever.

And, BTW, I will repeat this definition towards the end of this tome.

And, I will be giving discourses on meditation after every belt rank.

So, if you ever have question, get confused, or whatever, with these discourses, simply look here, or the section at the end of the book between Postures 88 and 89, and you'll be back on track.

Attention is fixing your awareness on something.

Meditation is holding your attention (on something) for a prolonged period of time.

Contemplation is holding your attention on something with the intent of perceiving it directly (as it is), and thus ridding yourself of separation from the object (your creation).

When you master meditation, in all its aspects, you achieve the illumination of direct perception (you become aware that you can be aware of something without the need for eyes, ears, and other physical tools.

The point here is to look out at the universe so intently that you are freed from mental machinations, and realize yourself as Awareness.

That is the definition, and I only want to say one thing: the meditations you will encounter in this book may be quite different, and especially described differently, than any other meditations you have ever encountered.

This is because I am not coming from the viewpoint of strictly yoga. I am coming from the fourfold viewpoint (Monk, Yoga, Martial Artist, Ascetic), and this expanded by work in various other fields, including my discoveries in Matrixing and Neutronics.

Bear that in mind as you progress, and worry not if you are already an accomplished Yogi, or accomplished in some other discipline.

I have seen the whole path, and I lead you rightly.

YOUR FIRST MEDITATION

Listen. Don't talk, don't wonder, don't look, don't do anything. Simply strike a pose, close your eyes, and listen.

You will find that your mind wanders. That's okay, just rein it in, shut it down, and...listen.

Listen to the world. Listen to the birds in the trees, the passing traffic. Listen to whatever passes through the universe of you.

Learn to listen during the white belt phase, and further meditations will be arriving at each belt level.

At various places during your practice you may experience uncomfortable phenomena.

Don't panic. No matter where you are, if you encounter something uncomfortable, simply listen. Listen until you are calm and once again at the center of your universe, then resume whatever meditation you were working on.

POSTURE ZERO
Prayer Position

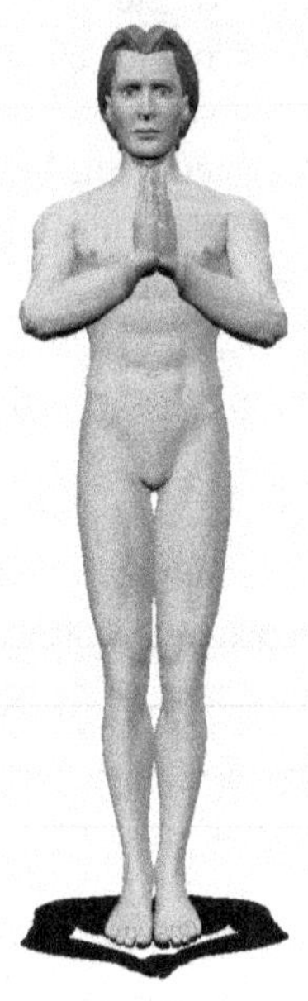

The Prayer Posture.
From this position do all others grow.

POSTURE ONE
Tadasana (Mountain Pose)

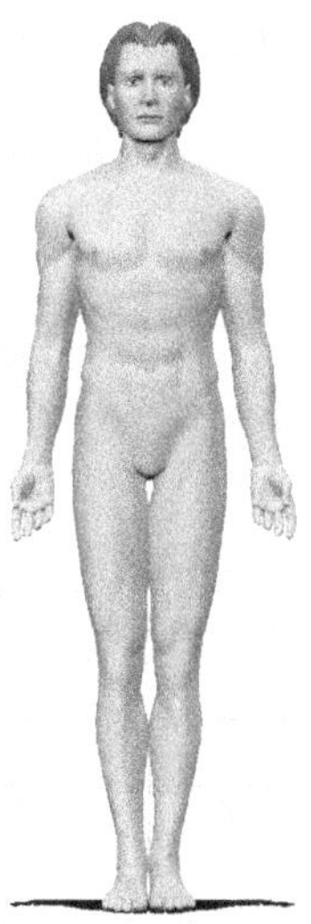

Feet together.
Shoulders slightly back.
Crown of head over pelvis.
Make sure pelvis is level.

Benefits sciatica.
Balances blood pressure.
Reduces insomnia.

There are many variations, including feet spread shoulder width, hands turned slightly, and so on.

Create yourself as a line perpendicular to the floor.

To progress, once you are stable, try closing the eyes and listening.

HOW THE BELT RANKING SYSTEM GREW

In the beginning, in the martial arts, there were supposedly only two rankings. White Belt and Black Belt. The words were Kyu (boy) and Dan (man).

To go from boy to man one had to mature. This didn't mean puberty, but rather a statement of the being, the attainment of a mature outlook, a degree of wisdom. A statement of 'I am.'

Unfortunately, the martial arts often became a rite of passage. This meant certain people were denied or otherwise put off the path.

Yoga is not concerned with a rite of passage, but steps leading to higher awareness.

As time went on, the number of belts in the martial arts increased. Sometimes valid, sometimes a selling ploy.

In the system I studied the belts were broken down to eight levels of 'boy,' but, actually, four colors. The colors were white, green, brown, and black.

White was the beginning: emptiness of experience. Snow in the fields where there was no growth.

Green was intermediate: the first shoots of spring, the first stage of growth.

Brown was advanced: the illusions of spring are gone, and the reality of fall arrived.

Black was expert: illusions of the real world are gone, and what is left is the person, the 'I am,' enduring through time. This was the truth of the spiritually aware being.

POSTURE TWO
Urdhva Hastasana (Upward Salute)

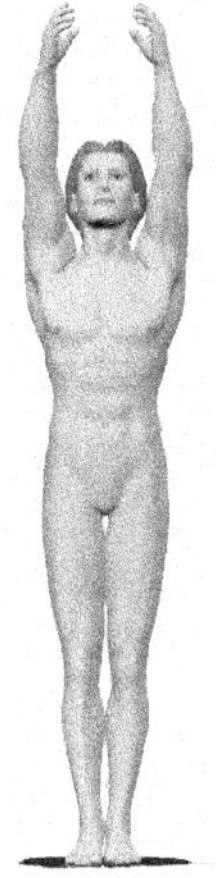

Reach upward.
Tilt the head slightly back and look up.

Lifts shoulders and ribcage.
Benefits shoulders and inner organs.
Again, many variations, including spread feet, arms together (prayer position).
And, when comfortable, close the eyes and listen. The world is not what you hear, it is what you are aware of.

Poses on right are 'leaning' mountain poses. It is quite enjoyable to alternate them, that is, to go from side to side and create 'vibration.'

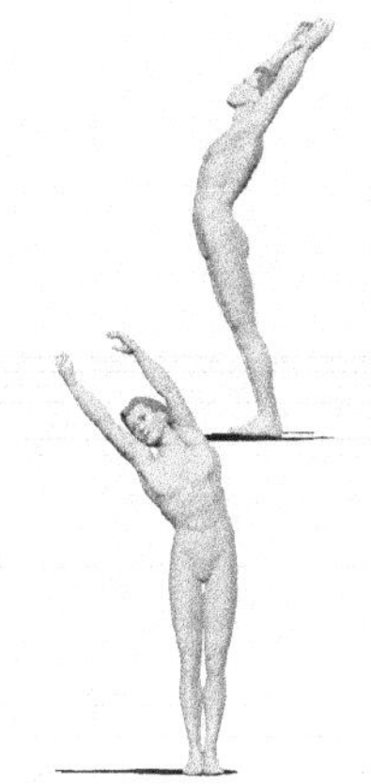

MOTION V NO MOTION

The universe is motion, it is good to study martial arts and create motion, analyze motion, manipulate motion, and so forth.

Yoga provides a starting point.

It is a Neutronic Principle: A point in all directions is no point at all.

This describes you as an Awareness

You don't exist in this universe, you are merely aware of it.

And you 'look' at it, and 'listen,' and so forth, by being aware through perceptic devices such as the eyes and ears and so on.

But you are not the perceptic devices, you are the Awareness looking through the perceptic devices.

I remember when I was three years old being very frustrated, laying in bed and trying to see behind me without using my eyes. I wanted my natural self back, I wanted to be aware, I didn't want to be trapped by flesh, unable to see everything; unable to see behind my head because I was limited to eyes.

So try it.

Be in pose, and see behind you without using your eyes. Be aware. Be all. Enjoy.

A point in all directions, you create the universe by manifesting light in all directions. You are the source, the awareness that cannot be perceived, and only another awareness can 'see' you. (Be aware of you).

POSTURE THREE
Utkatasana (Chair Pose)

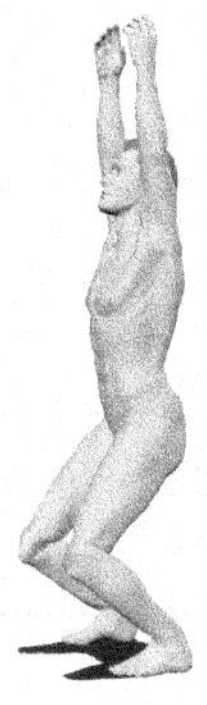

From the last pose…
Bend Knees
Tilt pelvis slightly.

Strengthens legs.

There is much variation on this pose, as one could bend forward and do the ski pose, or lean slightly forward (parallel lines between calves and arms, and so on. One could also create a routine.

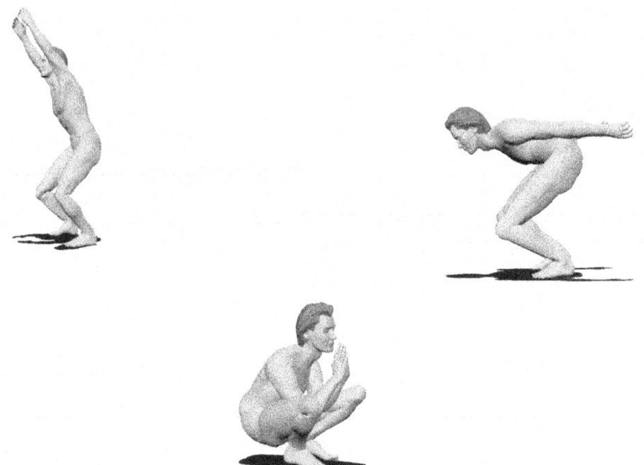

This 'squatting pose' makes for a wonderful routine. Simply go through the previous poses to this one, and back up again.

YOGA ROUTINES

In Yoga there are motionless poses, wherein one merely has existence, and observes the world, and thus creates more awareness.

There are also small routines, wherein one changes from one posture to another. These small routines are designed to bring awareness of the body in small increments. There are also large routines. The book, 'Yogata: The Yoga Kata,' is recommended as an example of a large routine. It covers all of Yoga, presenting the discipline from the larger viewpoint.

One can be a beginner to do The Yoga Kata, and work into the intermediate realm, which is what the form really is.

The nice thing is that one can see, as one travels through the large routine of The Yoga Kata, the many places where one can deviate and make an advanced and even expert routine out of the thing.

The point here is that by being motionless, one looks out, observes, becomes more aware, starts to ask questions like: who is looking? What am I, really?

By entering into slight motion one travels through the body, becoming more aware of the moving parts, learning how to adjust and fix it.

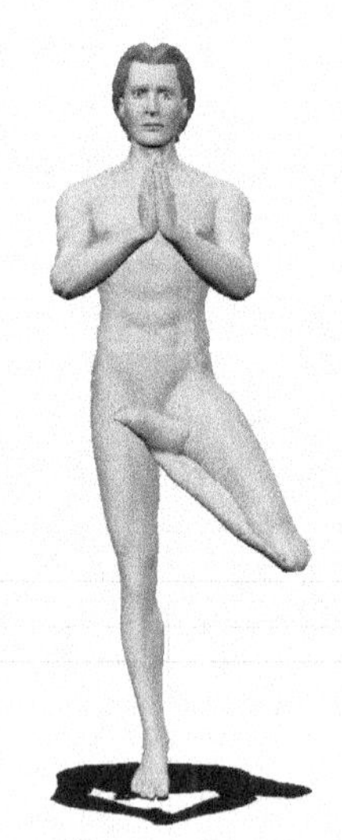

In the next section we will discuss how to matrix poses to find every single potential of motion, or non-motion, there is.

Relax. Breath. Enjoy.

POSTURE FOUR
Vrksasana (Tree Pose)

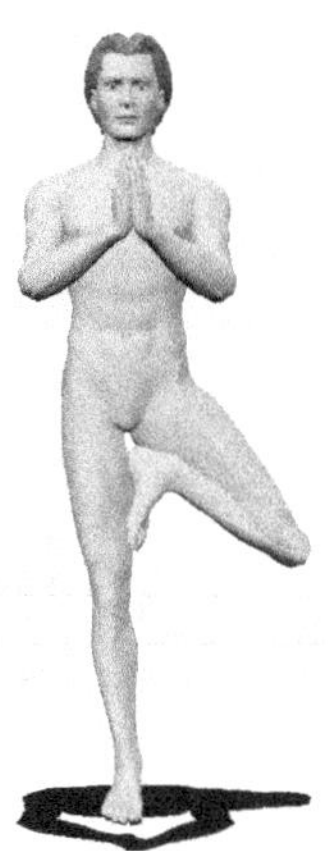

Time to go to one leg. Ten times more difficult to close the eyes, but ten times the benefit.

Strengthens legs,
opens the groin
stretches the inner thighs.

Closing eyes is twice as difficult now, but twice the benefits.

Some people prefer to lift the hands high, as if reaching for the sky.
I prefer the prayer, more difficult to stand, puts you in your head, makes you look at the world harder so as to hold yourself in position.

Examine the pose and its effects on your body, you don't need to hold it overlong, but you need to hold it long enough.

It may take a while to fold the foot, as in the pic to the right, maybe even some work on the Lotus posture, but you'll make it.

HOW LONG TO HOLD A YOGA POSE

This matter of how long you should hold a yoga pose is interesting.

In the martial arts, some stances we would hold for a minute or two, other stances we would practice what is called 'pile stancing,' where you hold the stance for hours.

This concept in mind, one can see how easy the transfer from martial arts to Yoga is, and, of course, the transfer from yoga to martial arts should be equally easy.

You see, when we pile stanced we improved by leaps and bounds. An hour in pile stance was better than an eight hour work out.

But to get back to Yoga and how long we should hold the stances, you need to become educated as to your body tolerances.

One can stand in a mountain stance for an hour. But if one stands in a tree stance for an hour there will be much pressure on the pelvis, and the sacroiliac. Thus, five minutes in tree might benefit the student and eliminate sciatica. However, six minutes might unbalance the 'joint' between the elephant ear bone and the triangle bone at the base of the spine, causing sciatica.

So it is a tricky road, because if you go a minute too far, you might end up with six months laid off, not to mention trips to the doctor.

Best to do a little, and watch the body for a day, then add a little more, and always err on the side of caution.

You don't want a broken body to get in the way of your learning how to focus your awareness.

To focus your awareness on pain is never fun.

POSTURE FIVE
Sukhasana (Easy Pose)

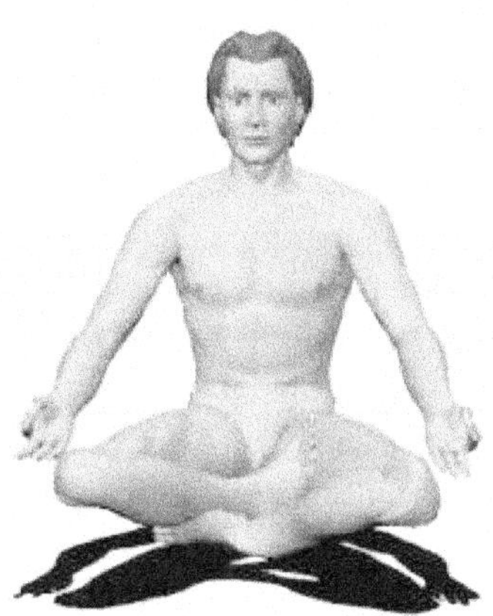

This is the Easy Pose.

The wrists should be forward on the knees, and you can see that the feet are a little weird. Still, everybody knows what sitting like an Indian means.

The reason this pose is slightly off is because the graphics program I am working with doesn't always bend the way it should. There are limits.

So the legs won't quite cross, and I had to bend the waist to make it look like he was sitting up and...and it doesn't matter if you get my meaning.

And, one might ask why didn't I use photographs?

Because they take memory.

If I used photographs for this book the memory would be so large that I would have trouble downloading it to the customer, would have to look into various programs for emailing large files, which might cost me security, and so on.

So I used the best program I could, and I saved memory so I could get the book to you.

SITTING IN CHAIRS

Some cultures don't have chairs, and they don't have much in the way of back problems.

People have to twist and bend their bodies to go up and sit down and cross the legs and...and all this opens the joints and adds strength to the legs.

Mind you, I am not saying to throw away your chairs, I am just saying to pay attention when you have been sitting at the computer too long, and stand up and stretch, maybe do a few squats, or lower yourself from the mountain pose and coil into a sitting pose facing the other way.

I said it before, and I'll say it again...don't underestimate the benefit of good, strong legs.

Legs, and feet especially, are loaded with trigger points. The mere act of walking sets the timing machinery for such things as heart beat and blood flow.

So strong legs equals strong heart, strong blood flow, and so on.

In fact, I think I've been sitting too long. Time to get up and stretch and contort and take a short walk. Maybe even yawn a little, and get all the systems to wake up. See you in a while.

POSTURE SIX
Garudasana (Eagle Pose)

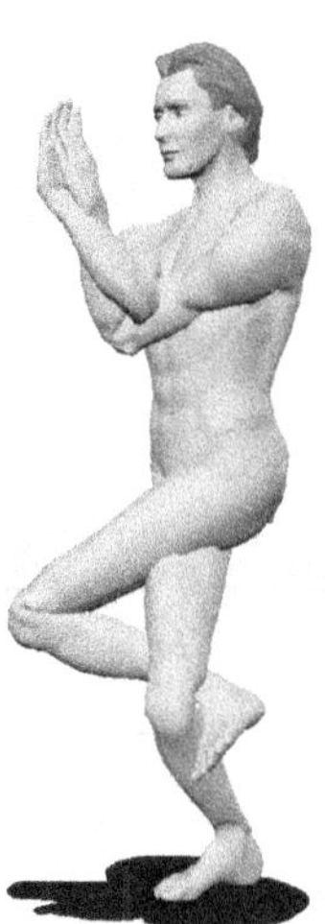

This is a fun pose, a mild twister, that will be easy to enter, but may take some time to get those last little 'clinchers' perfected.

Twisting like this, you will improve your body from ankle to shoulders and out to the wrists.

Mentally, you will gain an unwavering focus.

Make sure you tilt the pelvis forward. Tilting the pelvis forward always helps the hips, helps reduce and defeat sciatica, and makes for a balanced human being.

HOW TO MATRIX YOGA

Matrixing was originally developed in the martial arts, and it is a logical method for discovering all potentials of motion. Fortunately, it's pretty easy to use in Yoga, and will, again, no matter how subtle, explore all potentials of motion. Here is a matrix table.

	yes	**no**
yes	yes/yes	yes/no
no	no/yes	no/no

You may recognize it as a 'truth table' from Boolean Algebra. In that mathematics it is used to present three dimensional motion on a two dimensional surface. Such as, 3D on your computer screen. Or, plotting space flight on a screen.

What a truth table does, in matrixing, is present every possible potential of motion, and this by pairing every possible potential.

In the above examples, using only the two factors of yes and no, there are only four potentials. Thus, if one didn't know one of the potentials, by looking at the matrix one could instantly see the potentials, and would be able to say, 'Oh, I missed that one in the corner. Let me try it out and see if it works.

Obviously, some potentials won't work at all - you can't pick your nose with your elbow - but that's okay. Knowing that something doesn't work is just as important as knowing that something works. Often, more important.

We will leave the martial arts potentials for a later course in matrixing (I recommend Matrix Karate, as that was the first course in which I presented the science of matrixing, and it is loaded with goodies and basics and fun).

Here is how you make a matrix for Yoga.

	mountain	**tree**
mountain	mount/mount	mount/tree
tree	tree/mountain	tree/tree

Obviously mount/mount doesn't work.

You can go from mountain to tree, and from tree to mountain.

Tree to tree doesn't work.

Of course, if you switch legs, right to left, in a stance, then that changes the potentials and opens up the game, and mount/mount might work, and so on.

Okay, pretty simple, eh? You found which poses you can move into which poses, and you can practice those motions, and discover subtle, little things about your body.

So make a matrix for Mountain Pose and Lotus Pose (the famous crossed leg with the feet atop the thighs pose). You may come up with certain unworkabilities, but you can always go from Lotus to Lotus by switching which foot is on top.

But what is the motion involved in getting there?

Is there an intermediate stance you must or should do?

Do you have to do a lot of motion? A little motion?

Should you have your hands in the prayer stance to facilitate quick and easy switching? Yours arranged somehow else?

And so on.

Got it?

Good. Now draw a matrix with 100 yoga poses. That's only ten thousand potentials of motion you need to examine. Right?

Well, perhaps you should take a smaller number of poses.

Try making a list of poses for the belt level you are on. Take the first pose and matrix it with the second pose, then the third, and the fourth, and so on. Then use the second pose as your base and combine with all the poses of your belt level. Do this until all poses are matrixed. And you can matrix from belt to belt as you proceed through the system.

Many things won't work, and some will be so natural they are obvious, but there will likely be many that you never thought of. That's the glory of Matrixing.

POSTURE SEVEN
Plank Pose

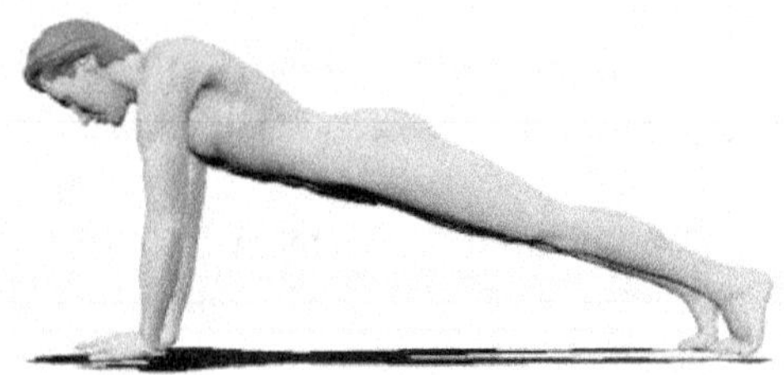

The Plank. Nothing more than a good, old push up, right? Well, sort of. The idea here is that you are not strengthening your arms so much as running (imagining) a stiff rod passing down your spine, energy globing in your shoulders. This will give you much energy, endurance, and strength.

So you could do push ups, but holding the stance for a period of time may have more benefit because you are imagining energy.

And, good news, there are lots of variations.

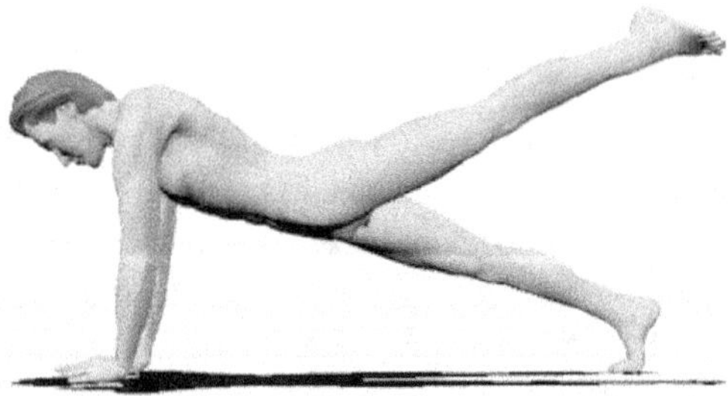

Do the plank while lifting one leg. This will strengthen the buttocks and back. Don't forget to alternate...you don't want to end up walking in circles because one leg is stronger than the other, do you?

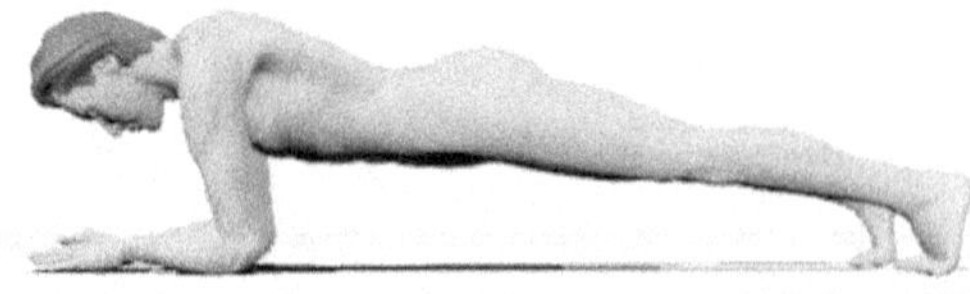

Here's a forearm plank pose, official term being the Dolphin Plank Pose.

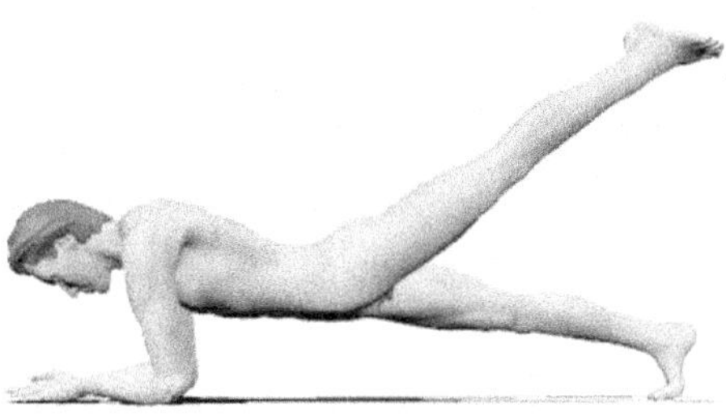

And here's the Dolphin Plank with a leg raise.

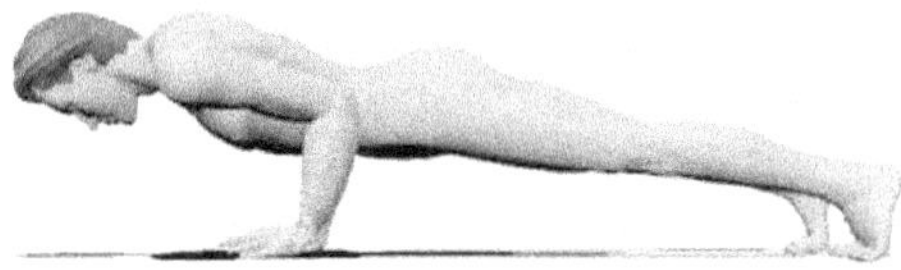

And a Chaturanga Dandasana (Four-Limbed Staff Pose).

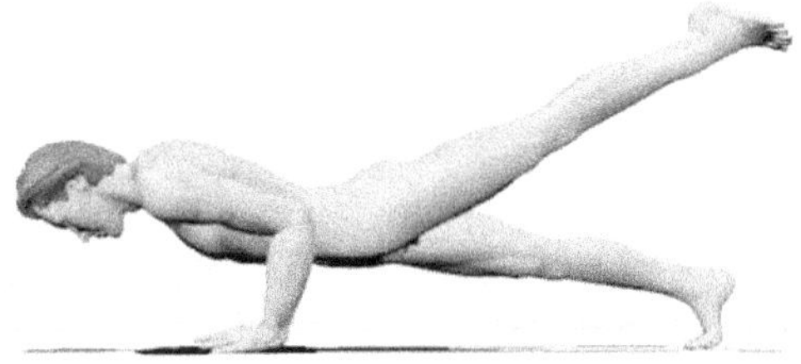

And a Chaturanga Dandasana (Four-Limbed Staff Pose) with a leg raise.

Do you see how many potentials you have here? Now write a matrix of these poses, and figure out how to get from one to other smoothly and efficiently. Explore the potentials of your body, and have a good time doing it.

YOGA ALIGNMENT

Aligning the body in Yoga is an interesting subject, with much opinion on either side of the fence. That said, one should explore both sides of the fence and find what suits them, what benefits them, what makes their expanse of skin glow with health and energy and spirituality.

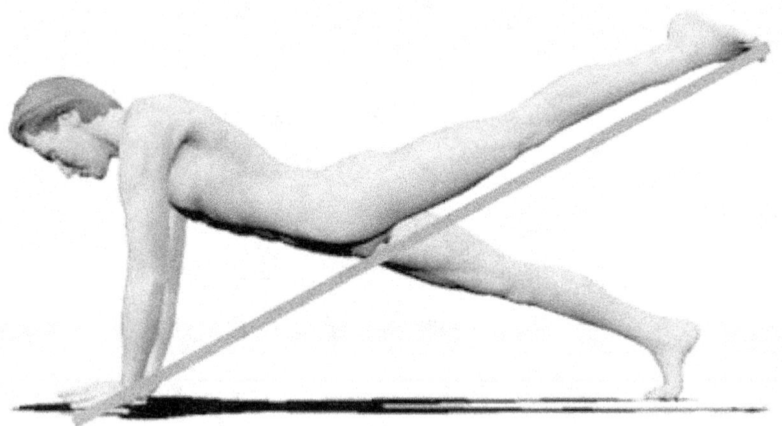

In the above illustration I have drawn a line.

Some people say the line should go from fingers to toes. Some people say the line should follow the axis of the leg and go to the center of the palm.

Some people say there should be no line, but rather the student should move the leg up to the extreme.

Now, there is MUCH argument for the extreme. I, however, prefer a geometrical approach, and I am always seeking lines that are parallel, that make Xs with exact angles, and so on.

I am not so much interested in contortionist as the perfection of thought that goes with a perfectly aligned body.

POSTURE EIGHT
Dolphin Plank Pose

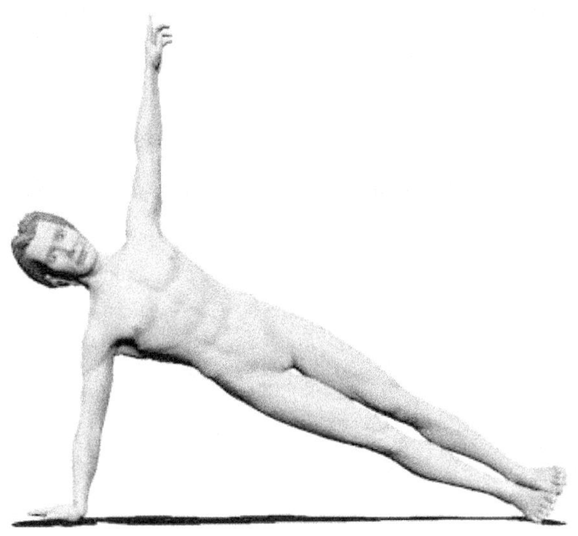

Here's a Dolphin Plank Pose. Excellent for shoulders and balance. When you strive for balance, remember, the muscles on both sides of the limb are going to fire quick and fast, these are the fast twitch muscles, and you will end up with a work out though you have done nothing more than twitch. Once you have the stance accomplished, and are experiencing no twitching, then you are going to work the deeper muscle, or the energy (prana, or chi) directly. And, of course, the mental aspect of this is incredible; you learn to focus awareness quickly and accurately.

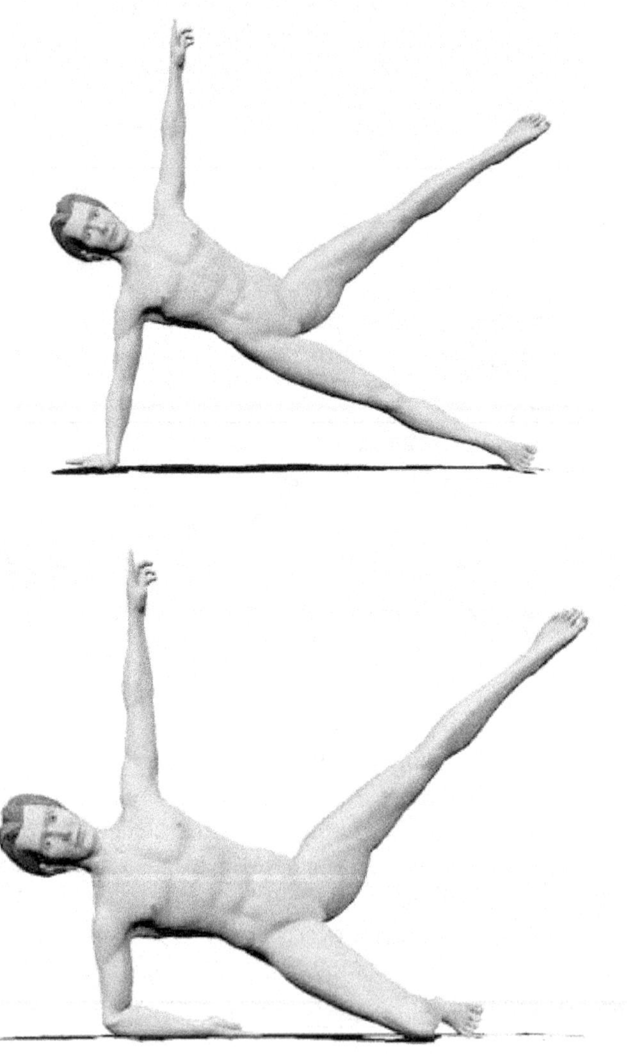

Feel free, when you are beginning, to modify the poses until you have built the strength and balance to do them.

One can bend the knee or the forearm, either separately or together (as in above posture), when doing this.

ALIGNING THE TAN TIEN

In the martial arts we call it the Tan Tien. It is a spot about two inches below the navel. In Yoga we refer to it as a chakra. This specific chakra is where body energy is created; it is the body energy generator.

To activate and flow power to the energy center, and thus energize your whole body, you should focus awareness on the tan tien. You do this by breathing as if to the tan tien. This is also called diaphragmatic breathing.

You don't really breath to the tan tien, air only goes to the bottom of the lungs. but this sets up a wave of energy that will course downward, below the lungs, and to the tan tien. Stand and breath in this manner and you will experience a tingling in your fingertips every time you breath deeply.

Another method you can use, more closely associated with Yoga, is to make the body alignment lines begin, end, or cross the tan tien. Do this first with your imagination, then make the pose do it.

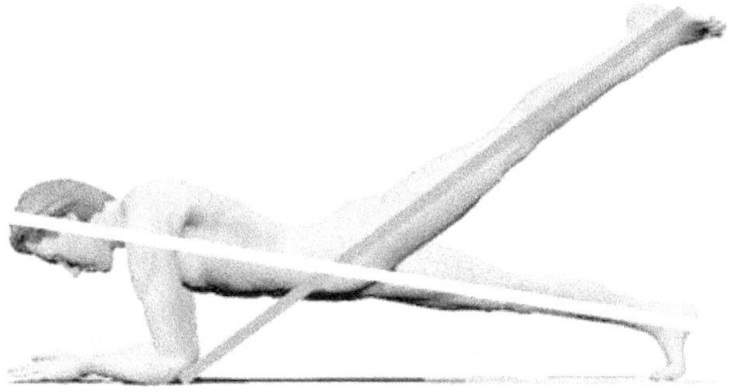

In the illustration above, the lines run through the tan tien.

There are many other types of geometry one can use in such endeavors as this, including circles and triangles and squares, and even such shapes as toruses and spirals.

POSTURE NINE
Purvottanasana (Upward Plank Pose)

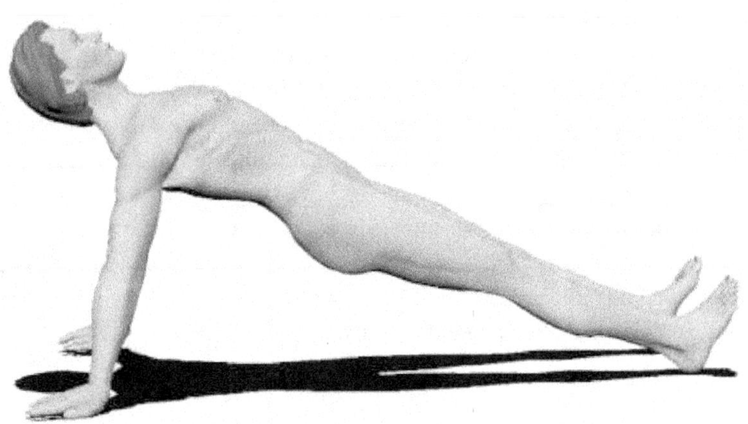

This is the upward Plank Pose. Obviously, you can run a little routine by going from plank to side plank to rear plank and back, or continue in that direction and do a complete revolution of the body.

And, you can figure out modifications of each pose to help you flow smoothly and easily.

The wrists and shoulders benefit from this pose greatly. Holding this pose for a length of time will greatly reduce fatigue as a factor of your life.

This pose also stretches the rib cage, which aids the internal organs.

Arching is very beneficial in this pose.

RELAXING

The most important thing you can do, when doing Yoga, is relax. If you use force, you make your body tense, and that is when you pull muscles.

Also, if you are tense then you are putting awareness into your muscles, and not...wherever you are supposed to be putting it.

There is a monstrous trap designed into Yoga, and I shudder to think how many free spirits have been abused by it.

Simply, think about it, by doing Yoga you think that you have to have Yoga to be a free spirit. Which is to say...you have to have a body.

Yikes!

A free spirit has no body!

Do you see the trap?

You are working to have no body, even as you implant within yourself the need to have a body. This is a very devious motor indeed.

Remember, a motor is two terminals between which there is tension (push/pull). The two terminals here would be the desire to not have a body, and the desire to have a body. And the tension between these two goals would keep you trapped in body for a long time.

Thus, relax as you do Yoga, forget about the body, even as you tell it to go into severe asana.

We don't break motors here, we simply understand them, and harness them, and discard them when we desire.

POSTURE TEN
Ananda Balasana (Happy Baby Pose)

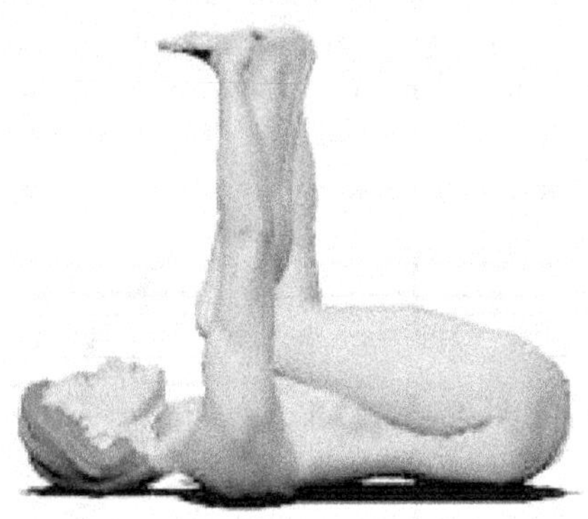

This is a wonderful pose for the hips. Indeed, not much else is happening here except the hips.

Well, there is the spine, that is relaxing, imagine the spine like water, a puddle spreading out on the floor, no tension within.

And, I hate to say it, but the brain relaxes. There is just something so joyful about this pose, and that is why babies do it.

Wah!

Grin.

You can use a belt to help position your feet in the beginning, if you need to.

THE DUALITY OF THE MOTOR

As stated, a motor has two terminals.

Now, one can assume a posture, and go to the next posture, and back again, and so forth, and one is simply creating and exercising a motor.

One can relax and find a more extreme posture, and thus make the motor function better. Or at least differently.

The interesting thing in Yoga is that we are translating push and pull into relax and relax.

You don't push the posture in one direction, you relax it in that direction.

You don't pull the posture in one direction, you relax it in that direction.

People who push or pull are creating a motor that will trap them.

People who relax are controlling that motor, and thus stepping out of that motor, and thus freeing themselves from that motor.

Apply this principle to everything you do in life. Find terminals which oppose, and cause them to relax, and, suddenly, the motor you have created becomes light and easy to manipulate.

It is especially fun to do this between two people who are at odds. It takes some wonderful imagination, but you will find that people actually love to be manipulated in this fashion. The reason? They love to experience freedom from the motors that entrap them.

POSTURE ELEVEN
Marjaryasana (Cat Pose)

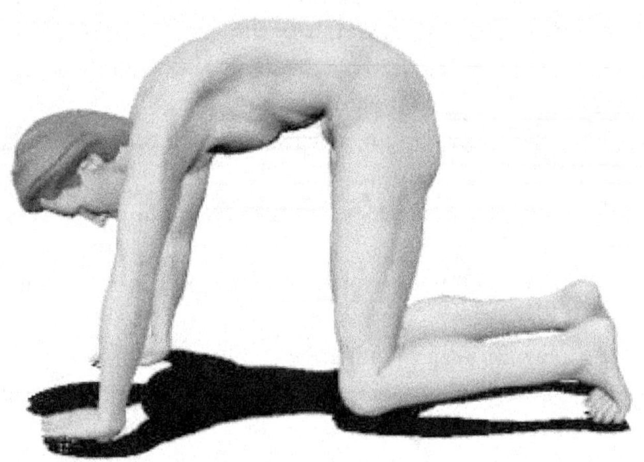

The Cat Pose is wonderful for flexing the spine, loosening it up, making it relax. You can alternate it with the next pose, called the Cow Pose.

Relaxing up, relaxing down, you stretch the limits of your body motor. Feels so-o-o good!

The organs like this gentle up and down motion, and you are loosening all those internal organs from their own machinelike stress.

Be gentle with your neck if you have an injury.

BTW, have you written out a matrix for the poses you know? Starting with a small list, and expanding it as you grow, is the best way to go.

FIXING THE MIND

I call it fixing the mind, for it does fix the mind, and that by the simple act of doing without it.

If you relax enough in pose, then you can fix your attention on something.

The mind is a bunch of memory, so by looking at something in the real world, you are not accessing the mind.

And why should you?

You should only call on the mind if you want to remember something.

It is a tool you should use, not be used by.

So focus your awareness on something.

If you are in a balancing pose, look at something in the world, triangulate, and assume balance, and lose your mind.

If you are in a posture which causes muscular tension, relax, look and the muscles and tell them to relax. Chances are, the only reason they were tense is because your mind told them to remember being tense...so now you can tell them to relax, and forget about any commands from the mind.

If you are practicing with eyes closed, look with your imagination. Look through the walls, through the mountains, and out to the far stars.

Your imagination is the flesh of your real body, you know. Not that body that you think you're in, but the stretch of how far you can extend awareness, and even through realms that have not yet begun to be.

Heck, that is how they become to be.

POSTURE TWELVE
Bitilasana (Cow Pose)

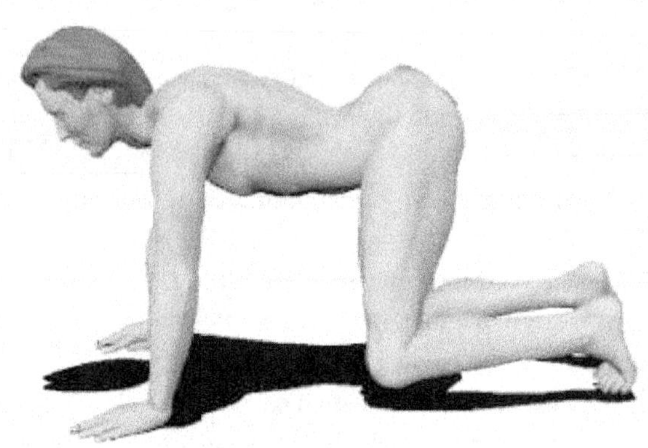

Relax, assume this posture by letting the belly sag. Imagine rubbing the floor with your belly.

You can look upward with this one, but make sure you are aggravating a neck injury. Neck injuries should do the pose as above.

This pose is designed to relax, totally and utterly, the internal organs.

Let those intestines sag, take all tension out of them, let them drag on all connections, and thus relax all and everything within the body.

It's amazing how good such a simple pose can make you feel.

And, I want to say something...too many people think Yoga is difficult, is contortionism.

No. It is relaxation. People who can do these simple poses are getting as much, maybe more, than somebody who is strenuously efforting at more difficult poses.

Yoga is not about how to tie the body in a knot...it is about how to untie the body from a knot.

So relax, affirm yourself, enjoy not working, be yourself, do Yoga.

WHAT THE UNIVERSE IS

I learned this rather quickly in the martial arts: to the degree that you are tense, to that degree you cannot move. And: to the degree that you cannot move, to that degree you are dead.

Life is Motion

Now, comes the question, what is the purpose of motion?

Well, you can move simply and sheerly because you want to, because you enjoy life.

And, even if you have no arms and legs, you can imagine motion. You can run energy through your body, and still find freedom.

The truth of the matter is that this universe is nothing but objects flying around, threatening to collide, having flow with potential force.

And, the next truth of the matter is that your body is a universe, with things flying around inside it, threatening to collide.

Can you make untense your body, so that whatever collisions happen within have no effect, are merely slippage asides rather than clunk and oh?

The body should be like liquid rubber, slithering against itself in never ending motion.

To do otherwise is to be concrete, to be something that collisions can lodge in and create damage.

To do otherwise is to hold disease and infirmity.

Wouldn't you really rather relax?

POSTURE THIRTEEN
Supta Padangusthasana (Reclining Big Toe Pose)

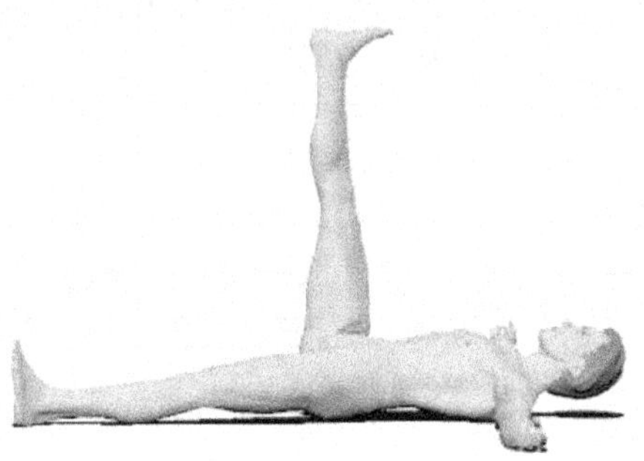

This is a great pose, good for stretching out the hips and groin.

Obviously, one can grab a belt and lace it around the foot and help raise the foot to the perpendicular position.

If the head is up, and slightly uncomfortable (like I have in the above pose) you should fold a blanket or put a thin pillow underneath the head, and practice relaxing down.

Now, the routine here would be to move the raised leg to one side, or the other, and touch it to the floor. Rest, breath, relax, and go to the other side.

This pose will stretch you, fix up the prostate gland, sciatica, improve digestion, and all sorts of other things. One must never underestimate how much benefit can be had by having the legs in good working order.

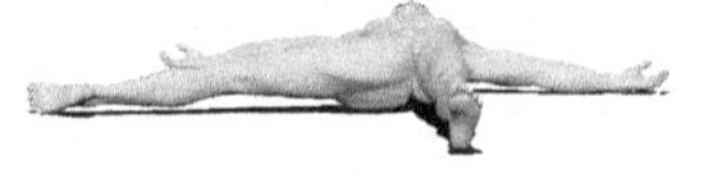
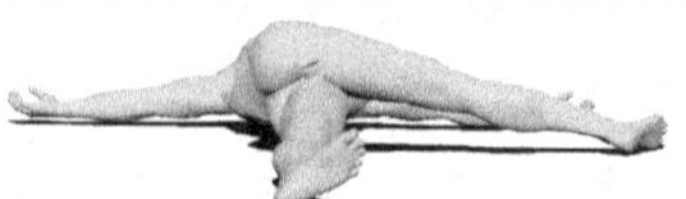

Here are the two poses where you move the Big Toe raised leg to one side or the other.

If you have trouble with this, a great way to start is by doing it with a bended knee.

Breath. Relax. Enjoy

WHERE MATRIXING AND NEUTRONICS CAME FROM

In 1974 I achieved Black Belt. Over the space of several months I had several realizations, my life changed, and the way I conducted my life really changed.

You can read about the things I went through, and many of these realizations in other works I have written on the Martial Arts. Entering the Third Level is probably one of the more significant books, though it may be hard to find.

However, this isn't martial arts, and we are getting ahead of ourselves. What we need to do is discuss only certain data concerning the human experience.

The exact realization I had, when I achieved black belt, one that is universal and quite compatible with where you are on the road to enlightenment, is...

> For something to be true,
> the opposite must also be true.

This is actually a verbalization of the yin yang, and quite potent. You can work this sucker around and come up with all sorts of martial arts strategies and principles and concepts and so on.

The main thing, however, is that it defines a motor.

Remember, a motor is two terminals between which there is tension (push/pull).

There is a motor in a cell, in an atom, in a big corporation, in a wing...in everything.

And everything is a motor.

Did you expect the minutia of a universe to be the opposite of the universe itself?

Did you expect all the little motors not to reflect the big motor?

Let me tell you, whatever you believed...the opposite is true. Grin.

So the universe is built of something (hard light/hard chi/hard prana/ hard whatever) but it is still built of light/chi/prana/something.

And this hard something (hard light/hard chi/hard prana/hard whatever) is built of light something (soft light/soft chi/soft prana/soft whatever).

So the universe is a motor built of hard and soft, something and nothing, things and...no things. Or nothing.

Now, I stumbled across matrixing while I was trying to figure everything out. And after I matrixed enough things, I arrived at nothing...or spirituality.

The body is something, and the human being is...nothing, which is to say it is awareness, which can't be measured, and is therefore nothing.

The funny thing is that when you read sacred texts, which is to say books that were written and lasted over long periods of time, this is what they say.

In the beginning God created the heavens and the earth. (The Bible)
The nameless is the origin of Heaven and Earth. (The Tao)

Heaven and earth, as mentioned in these epistles, are two terminals to a motor.
To mention just two such ancient manuscripts.

And, to reverse engineer a bit, what is God?
God doesn't exist in this universe (can't be named, is nameless, etc.)
The only thing that cannot be seen (or even measured even scientifically) in this universe is...awareness.
God is Awareness.
You are Aware.
Therefore you are god. At least, some part of the Greater Awareness to which, through Yoga, we join.

Do you understand how vital it is that you become loving and compassionate and forgiving and so on? Simply, you are the one creating all the wars and diseases and so on, and we really need to end all that. And we can. By making every single being Aware.

POSTURE FOURTEEN
Balasana (Child's Pose)

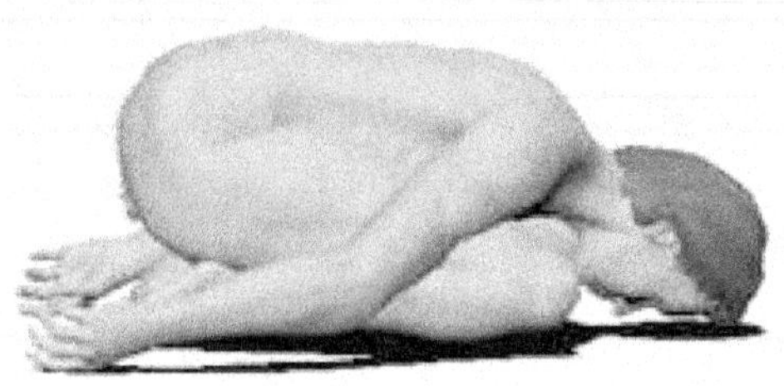

This a very relaxing pose, often called a 'restorative' pose.

I find it very enjoyable to grab the heels (a modified Rabbit Pose), and just rest. After a good work out you are always supposed to cool down with a restorative pose. These moments are always very enlightened moments. You'll find yourself having thoughts that gently change you. You'll find yourself deep in wonder, far away in a meditative universe, and then suddenly back in the real world.

These moments are to be treasured.

To not do a restorative pose after a work out is to deny yourself the icing on the cake.

Always, always, always end a work out with a restorative pose, and enjoy those moments of oneself with yourself to the max, for they are the truth of you coming to light.

They represent what Yoga is all about.

EXPLORING THE MATRIX OF THE BODY

Matrixing is based on a graph which will help you find every potential of motion.

In Yoga, the matrix can be reduced down to the simplicities of X, Y, and Z.

In algebra X goes side to side, Y goes up and down, and Z goes to and from (depth).

When you move the body through space, in the martial arts, while this provides a basis for movement, one will find there are a lot more geometries to be explored.

When you move the body in Yoga you make the body taller or shorter, move it side to side, and...twist it.

We are not stick figures on a piece of paper, you see, and we can move back and forth, but as Yoga takes place in a relatively small space, Z becomes a twist, a rotation, a revolution.

This is an interesting concept to ponder, so think of it this way. You are in a cube, and you can only go so far in a cube, and then you must bounce off the walls (the extent of your reach) and turn...or twist.

Now, one could label this whole phenomena differently. We can't levitate (at least, that's not in the lesson plan of this book), so we are on the floor, which would mean that Y is truncated, and each dimension (X, Y, and Z) has the potential for a twist...but all that's not important. All that is important is that you can stretch in any direction only so far, and then you start to twist.

Mathematics of the human body aside, think of it this way: to twist is to wring the body out.

Now we're talking!

POSTURE FIFTEEN
Savasana (Corpse Pose)

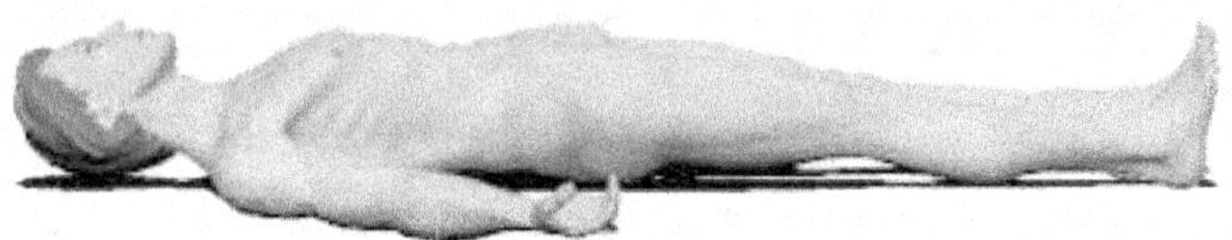

This is the big restorative pose. Simply lay on your back and let your body puddle into the ground, and let your thoughts puddle to wherever they will go.

A good yoga session, a good restoration, and your life is going to fly!

ORANGE BELT

The second belt is an orange belt. I have explained about the concept of seasons as one progresses towards awareness in the martial arts. Another theory is of the spectrum. Simply, one goes the full spectrum of personal development, as represented by the full spectrum of color.

Now, in the four belt scheme of things, there are four colors: white, green, brown, and black.

We would make smaller belt levels by putting tips on the belts, or by running a strip along the length of the belt.

Thus, we wound up with…

White.
White with a green stripe.
Green.
Green with a white stripe.
Green with a brown stripe.
Brown.
Brown with a white stripe.
Brown with a black stripe.
And Black.

And there are several levels of black, which we will not bother with in this tome.

In more commercial systems, ones which followed the spectrum concept of belt colors, the belts were…

White.
Orange/
Purple.
Blue.
Green.
Brown.
3rd Brown. (one tip)
2nd Brown. (two tips)
1st brown. (three tips)
And, several levels of black.

So the colors were arranged in different ways, were different, and so on.

But brown belts were brown, and they had three levels, and that was pretty much set in stone.

In this book, 'Black Belt Yoga,' we will use...

White.
Orange.
Purple.
Blue.
Green.
Brown.
Black.

Obviously, poses will get more difficult, instructions will remain simple, but hard to follow, and you will have fun.

YOUR SECOND MEDITATION

This is the OM Meditation.

To understand OM, you could do several years of Karate and learn how to do the Kiai, and then translate that particular vibration into a word, like OM, and hold it in meditation.

But, since beginnings are probably where we are, perhaps you have a shower stall? Or a friend with a shower stall. (Oh, the look you are going to get when you head over to Bertha's house and ask to use her shower stall!)

Stand in the shower and say OM.

Let it drag out a bit.

Find the place in the shower stall where all the echoes seem to come back to you. It will sound hollow, and there will be an actual vibration.

You may have to go up and down the scale a few times to find it, and move around, but it is there, and when you find it it will be unmistakeable.

Incidentally, I happen to be a hearing aid dispenser, and in the course of my studies I came across several interesting acoustic phenomena concerning sound, and this is what prompted me to describe this method for finding the one sound that is OM.

To go on, Once you have found this sound, go home and sit in simple pose like the Easy Pose or the Lotus Pose-you want to be balanced when you first do this-and create the OM sound.

Later, you can play with other postures, but be aware, you can cause ill effects if you do this in the wrong posture. Body positions create different harmonics, and you may find OM uncomfortable, and even repulsive, in some postures.

Best advice is to stick with the balanced easy style postures.

Generate the OM, low and soft, and let it ring. Let it vibrate.

As you generate OM, listen to how the vibrations act as they encounter the world around you.

You are like a bat sounding the world.

But, do OM long enough, and the world is going to take on different characteristics. Vibrations will charge the world around you.

And, you may be freaked out the first time OM changes the color of something, or moves something.

Don't be freaked, merely continue, and all will right.

And, you will discover that you are a voice without a body.

POSTURE SIXTEEN
Baddha Konasana (Bound Angle Pose)

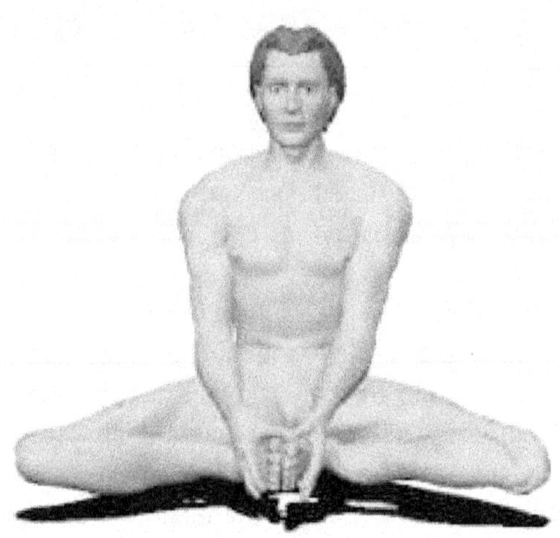

This is a wonderful pose for opening the hips. Simply place the soles of the feet together, grasp with your hands, and relax.

The hips are interesting joints. They have a ball and socket, but there is also the sacroiliac 'joint.' The sacroiliac is the elephant ear bone and the bottom triangular spinal bone (sacrum and ilium).

Some people say this isn't a joint because it doesn't move. But it does move, else we wouldn't have a sacroiliac slip, and the accompanying sciatica, and so on. And, of course, there is much belief that the sacroiliac can't slip unless the spine is first out of alignment.

The reason I tell you this is not to give you a course on anatomy, but to encourage you to explore anatomy on your own. Get medical charts, examine the skeleton and the blood vessels and the organs and everything that you can. The more you know, the less mysterious will the world be...and the faster you will progress in yoga.

THE PATANJALI

We have spent a little time discussing matrixing, and a bit of time concerning ourselves with Neutronics. This has been useful, as you will see in future pages, but I know it can be frustrating. After all, such subjects, and subjects like the martial arts, may seem a bit removed from the practice of Yoga.

But, remember, we are taking a more holistic viewpoint, attempting to understand all four paths and how they mesh. And these subjects we have discussed will come in handy in the short later on. But, for now, let's step to the side a bit. Let's discuss something called Patanjali.

Before we discuss, let me say that there is a dearth of material on the belief systems that surround good Yoga. This is because the material (sacred scripts) have been twisted through translation and culture and whatnot or the millennium.

But how can you progress if you don't know where you are going?

How can you understand the experiences of the spirit you are undergoing as you travel down the yogic road?

The Patanjali is the prime text when it comes to instruction manuals for Yoga. It describes much concerning the spirit and how it works.

Unfortunately, as I said, this text has been mangled by transmission through culture and time and language and all those other sorts of silly things that make up this concept called evolution.

In the Patanjali, we are talking real evolution.

Not the traceries of mankind as he wiggles across his time on earth.

Patanjali himself was born about 150 BC. Born, or perhaps that was the approximate time he compiled the sutras, or verses, of Yoga.

Specifically, he compiled four books, one of which he is said to have written himself.

Now, the study of Yoga is much older, but Patanjali's collection of Sutras are significant, for the verses became able to be studied as a single collection, as a single body of knowledge...and thus could be applied to the practice of Yoga to an unprecedented degree. And they are powerful verses indeed.

The four books of Patanjali are:

Samadhi Pada - which describes how to 'join' with the one (Greater Awareness).

Sadhana Pada - which describes two forms of Yoga, including the famous 'eight-limbed yoga.'

Vibhuti Pada - which deals with the manifestation of certain abilities through a practice of Yoga, and why these abilities (powers) should actually be avoided.

Kaivalya Pada - which describes the liberation of the non-physical 'I am.'

I have offered neutronic translation of the Patanjali elsewhere, and it will probably be made available at ChurchofMartialArts.com, so how deep we shall go into this subject remains to be seen.

The most important thing is to de-taint the sutras, to fix the manglings of language and culture and such, so that the meanings can be properly delved.

This depends, of course, upon understanding Neutronics and the real nature of the universe.

That's enough for now. Let's asana.

POSTURE SEVENTEEN
Virabhadrasana II (Warrior II Pose)

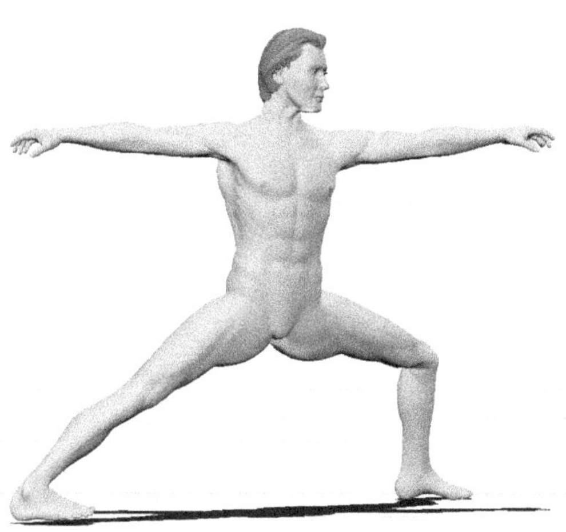

It is actually easier to do Warrior II before you do Warrior I. That's okay. In the long run it doesn't matter, and neither of the Warrior I and II poses is much more difficult than the other.

That said, one should stare forever. Stare as if looking through the walls, the trees of the forest, the very mountains. Stare as if you are looking right off the horizon of good, old planet Earth and into the forever.

Imagine you are seeing right through the end of the universe, and right into God's big, blue eye.

God doesn't have two eyes, only one. It (God) is not dualistic, as in man and woman, and certainly doesn't require two halves of a body. God is one body. One awareness, no sides, no favoritism, no blinking.

Do this asana long enough and you will be not just a warrior, but a God.

ENTERING PATANJALI

The first book of the Patanjali has to do with becoming spiritually conscious. That is, to be aware of yourself as a spiritual being, and in a spiritual universe.

Interestingly, one of the first points made is that one should control their psychic nature. That is, to be in control of that which is mysterious, invisible, etc. Do you understand how oblique this instruction is?

To do this you have to understand that you are awareness, and that you are looking through the perceptics (eyes, nose, ears, etc.) the human body.

Okay, this is fine. But comes the question, what gets in the way of the psychic nature?

What gets in the way is your mind.

In the Japanese there is an expression, 'mushin no shin,' which means, 'mind of no mind.' Literally, you must have a mind that does not rely on the mind.

The mind is just a bunch of memory.

So you must live your life without being distracted by the mind.

In other words, you must see reality as it is, and not through the filter of the mind.

Sounds complex, eh?

No.

Simply look at reality, and don't be distracted.

When you are in a pose, don't start thinking about the time Aunt Matilda smacked you upside the head. And every time you do start to think about dear, old Auntie...refocus on reality.

Look at a tree, a spot on the wall, listen to the sounds, but every time you find your focus wandering, and yourself thinking of other stuff, realize it and go back to focusing your awareness on what is.

The now and the here. Nowhere. That is the secret of enlightenment.

Everybody else is asleep.

People who see what is now and here...they are awake.

POSTURE EIGHTEEN
Virabhadrasana I (Warrior I Pose)

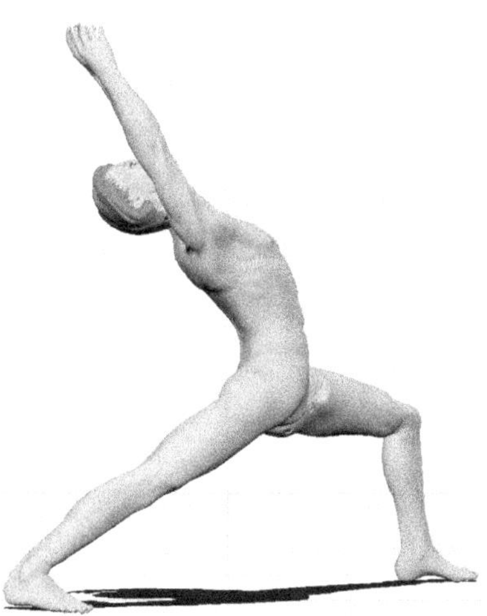

Warrior I is one of those iconic yoga poses. It also represents the front stance in many martial arts.

Doing this pose works nearly every body part. The specifics I enjoy are balance, strong legs, and far sightedness. It is delightful to stare upwards, and suddenly realize that you are seeing a lot more than you thought.

This is one of those poses you can do for a long time, and get nothing but benefit.

Many people prefer to do it with the arms and torso straight up. I prefer the bent back version. I love the gentle spine work of this stance.

As gentle as this pose is, be careful if you have high blood pressure or heart problems.

Relax. Breath. Enjoy.

THE FIVE PSYCHIC ACTIVITIES

There are five activities that Patanjali warns us against. Remember, these are the activities attributed to the spirit that get in the way of us realizing ourselves as spirit...as awareness.

First is not being wise. Or, being immature. This is the cruelty, you get a body, you are young, dumb and full of...stuff, and you do dumb things. Things that will retard your spiritual growth. Maybe you steal a car, maybe you don't keep your word, but there are all these things that people who are young do that they shouldn't. Best way out of this is just to study concepts of virtue...and do yoga. Pick a virtue and let your mind wander on it while in pose. Not a difficult pose, just an Easy Pose, or a Lotus Pose, or a Tree Pose. A White Belt or Orange Belt pose from this book will usually do the trick.

Second, self interest. So many people make decisions based on how it will benefit them, and not how it will benefit others...and all.

As a body you might have a specific self interest, getting the fastest car. As a spiritual being you might choose a vehicle that gets good mileage, carries lots of people, and that sort of thing. A car is nothing more than moveable space, after all.

Good mileage uses less gas which helps the planet. Carries more people (or stuff) is efficient and gets more work done.

So which is better for everybody?

One of the interesting concepts to be discovered, especially in the martial arts, but which should carry over to Yoga, is in the word Samurai. The meaning of the word Samurai is 'to serve.'

Stopping thinking about yourself, and start thinking about how you can help other people. You will find yourself joining the Greater Awareness before you know it.

Third, lust. You want sex, kink, experiences that waken the sausage (or make wet its dainty, little counterpart), and do little for the good of mankind. You hide in a room and masturbate, instead of working for the common good. You have lustful thoughts concerning innocent maidens, instead of making a well balanced family.

Do you see the imbalance here?

The point is that you are not flesh, and you shouldn't be trapped by the flesh, and lust is definitely a trap.

If you find yourself having impure thoughts, do an asana, a difficult one that requires muscles and balance. If that fails, take a long hike, run, lose yourself in the woods. Or, take a cold shower.

Fourth, hate. You are an I am. He (her) who you hate is an I am. Do you understand that you are just hating yourself? Hating the other part of you that lives in the Greater 'I am' Awareness? How can you join the Greater Awareness if you hate it?

That's like saying, "I'm going to run a mile, but hate my legs while doing it. Man, it wouldn't be but a few yards before your legs were tired and unable to continue the race.

Refresh yourself, rejoice in yourself, give up black thoughts.

If you do find yourself hating, force yourself to go to that (who) you hate and do something for them.

Obviously, do not do this if the other person is dangerous to be around. Do your benefits from afar in that case, think your kind thoughts from many miles away.

Fifth, attachment. This is very neutronic. Remember, a motor is two terminals between which there is tension (push/pull). Thus, do not enter into motor with the universe, or the things of the universe. Do not become a terminal for something in the universe. Do not think you HAVE TO HAVE that faster car, that brighter shade of underwear, that new house.

The way out of this trap is simply to live frugally. Buy a house with just a couple of rooms, and those for specific purpose. Don't fill it with junk, but rather cots for sleeping, and bricks and boards for bookshelves, and so on. Learn how to be compact in your living, how to get along with others in confined spaces.

Remember, to be in motor (to attach yourself) to the universe is to be the universe. Better to be you, an Awareness that cannot be measured by the universe. That is spirit, and that is truth.

POSTURE NINETEEN
Adho Mukha Svanasana (Downward-Facing Dog)

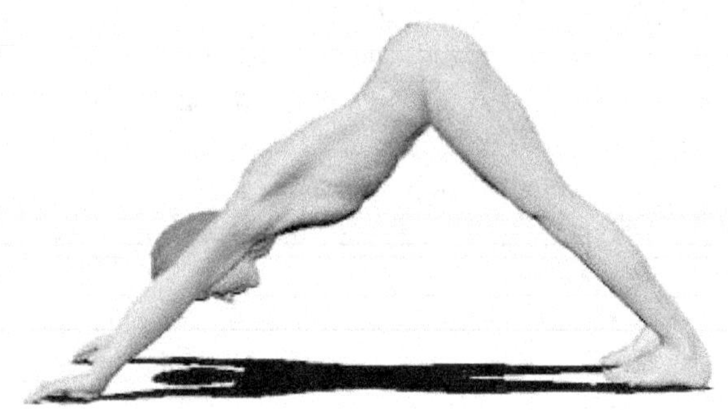

Another iconic Yoga asana. This is a fold at the waist, with the hands and feet flat upon the ground.

It is easy to do this pose, difficult to hold it at exactly 90 degrees with the feet flattened out.

This pose energizes and stretches, improves digestion, relieves headaches, is good for high blood pressure.

The real joy is in the stretch in the back. Difficult to do perfectly, but the wonderful sensations that calm you and energize you when you finally make it.

To the right is a Downward Facing Dog with a leg raise. Practice alternating the raises right and left.

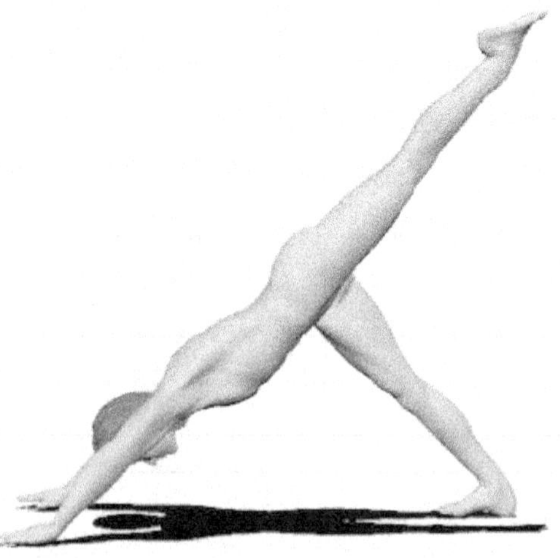

Relax. Breath. Enjoy.

ANOTHER VIEWPOINT OF THE FIVE PSYCHIC ACTIVITIES

The five psychic activities-which are often referred to as 'mental activities,' though that is not entirely accurate-are being too scientific, not being logical, not understanding why the universe is, trapped by dreams (fantasies), trapped by memory.

Now, the first two are interesting, because they seem to contradict. Being too scientific, not being logical. But being scientific means you are obsessing on measuring the universe. Not being logical refers to reasoning. So they don't really contradict.

So be scientific, but don't obsess on it, be willing to bend the universe as you need to. This is not too difficult, and you will realize this as you become more liberated.

And, be logical. Observe the universe, and specifically the beings living in the universe, and learn to predict their behavior. Learn what action leads to what other action.

What type of man will lie to a beautiful girl?

What type of girl will forsake love for cash, no matter the divorce.

What type of child is a whiner and needs a strong hand, and what type of child is gentle, and needs to be encouraged?

I prefer to think of the universe as something that can be strictly measured, and human beings something that you apply logic to. Though, to be honest, this is not always true, and the mix and match can often be confusing.

Number three is fascinating, for imagine being an animal in a zoo, and not knowing what bars are. Yet, that is the predicament of mankind. If he can just realize that he made his own invisible bars, that the universe is as he constructed it, then he will be liberated right then.

The truth is that the universe is a place you made up to have your existence in...then it got a little out of control, and started controlling the creator. Talk about your basic Frankenstein Complex. Sheesh!

Number four is dreams, fantasies. Isn't a person who is living a dream or fantasy asleep, just to be having such a dream or fantasy?

So, WAKE UP!

Don't live your life according to the dictates and conditions of false realities.

So simple, yet who has the power and the strength and the endurance and the vision to sit in pose and listen...and therefore awake?

Persistence, my friends. That is the key. And when you think you have failed, simply persist some more.

Number five is memory. Memory is a false reality, for it is a reality that has already happened, so why do you conduct yourself according to what has already happened, as opposed to what is actually happening?

I am fond of telling people that if they have reaction time, they are acting because of something that has happened before, and this has caused a gap in their awareness.

I am also fond of wondering why people cry, or have other unpleasant emotion, after something has happened. It has already happened! It is done!

This last, incidentally, is how I defeat unpleasant memories attempting to move me. I have the memory pop up, and I realize that it is not a pleasant memory because I start to feel bad, so I simply say to myself, "That is past. That's all done."

I immediately feel better, and the memory goes away fast, and it loses its power over me.

POSTURE TWENTY
Urdhva Mukha Svanasana (Upward-Facing Dog)

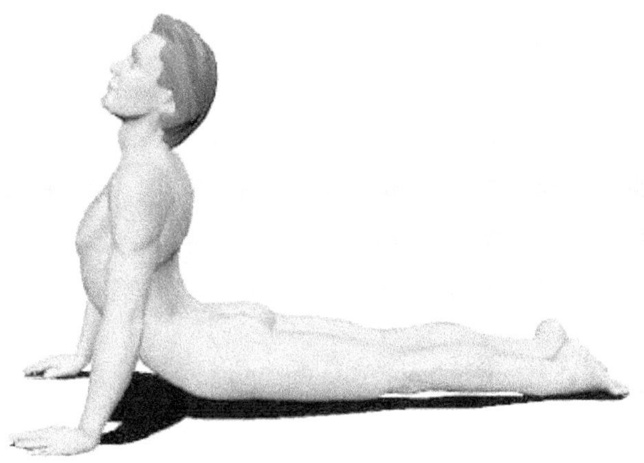

From the Plank position, sag the belly and look upward.

Some people prefer looking slightly downward, and perhaps this is good advice for the beginning, but, eventually, you want to look up. That's in the name of the pose, after all.

Now, this pose will stretch the body, strengthen the shoulders, and make you feel pretty darn good. Just take it easy in the beginning.

Also, I am fond of telling people that if they bend one way, they should balance that bend by doing a bend in the other direction.

Many people have back problems because they are always bending forward. Bending back, as in this pose, will reverse much damage, but you have to be careful, especially when starting. You don't want to overdo anything and cause damage.

DON'T FORGET TO MATRIX

I talk about matrixing and Neutronics, lead you into Patanjali, and we must not forget to Matrix.

Remember, start with a couple of simple poses, combine them for all potentials, and move on.

Hopefully, these small bites have resulted in you matrixing all the White Belt poses. If not, don't worry, it's never too late to go back and start looking and doing.

Now, as you learn an Orange belt pose, work it, and start going back through the white belt poses.

And, start combining it with the orange belt poses.

You should be doing this with each new belt of material you get.

Yes, it may take some time, but you will be discovering things that people with lifetimes in Yoga have never figured out.

And, more important, you will be figuring out how to make a mistake, and how to avoid it, and what to do about it, and all sorts of other things.

Dealing with mistakes, being able to live with your mistakes in the first place, and make them into something more than mistakes, that is the best education you can possibly have.

Now, that all said, one of my favorite routines is to:

Lay down in a Child's Pose.
Go to a Cat's Pose
Go to a Cow's Pose.
Go to a Dog Faces Downward Pose.
Go to a Dog Faces Upward Pose.
Go to a Plank Pose.
Go to a Dog Faces Upward Pose.
Go to a Dog Faces Downward Pose.
Go to a Cow's Pose.
Go to a Cat's Pose.
Return a Child's Pose.

A simple routine, it will vibrate your back like a violin string, giving it immense good health.

You can start with simpler routines, maybe just the cat and the cow, or the up and down dogs, but eventually you want to be able to do this one, and even add to it.

POSTURE TWENTY-ONE
Prasarita Padottanasana (Wide-Legged Forward Bend)

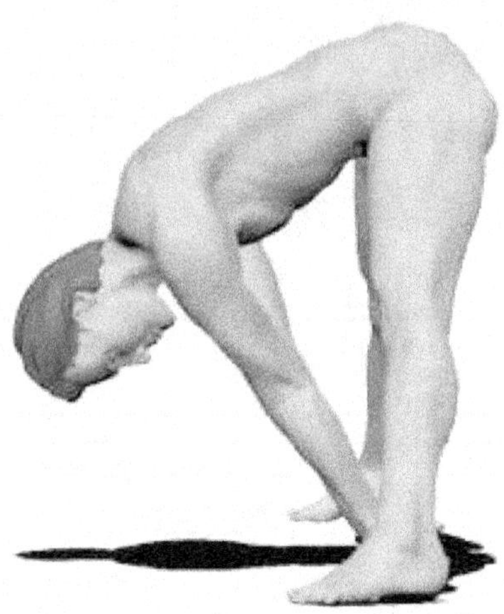

The wide-Legged Forward Bend will start you off on folding at the waist. While this one is easy, you'll find that later incarnations are difficult. When you reach the Big Toe Pose you'll be glad you spent time on this one.

The key to this is not to bend the back, but to fold the waist.

To bend the back is to cause undue pressure on the bones in the spine.

Fold deep, and pull on the ground back between your legs.

To fold at the waist is to learn how to relax the thighs, and to bend oneself all-l-l the way over. Very beneficial to stretching the legs through spine, and helping the kidney and liver.

Be careful if you have low back problems. Strengthen the back through other poses before trying this one.

BREATHING

I should have gone into this before, but...so much to talk about if you are going to get truly educated.

There are many methods for breathing, especially as one travels through the various asanas.

In the martial arts the main breathing is to breath from the center (tan tien-located an inch or two below the navel). Breath out when you expand the body, and in when you contract the body.

In Yoga, this advice can be followed.

However, you should relax the body, forget the body, and breath out through the hands, when you are stretching. Let your breath become intention, let your body relax into your intention, and no posture will elude you.

Sometimes you should focus on a body part, this puts energy into the body part. Examine the poses you are doing and where you are trying to go with the pose before doing this type of breathing.

Remember, prana means breath, and it is a life giving force.

There is prana in the universe, what martial artists call chi, or ki, and there is life giving force in your body, but it all comes down to awareness.

Direct your awareness, and that is like a 'prana light,' or 'chi light,' giving energy.

Awareness is everything, you must learn to focus your awareness direct your awareness, expand your awareness...you must learn awareness and how it works for every geometrical form in the universe.

In the beginning, you focus awareness by breathing. That moves energy, and suddenly you realize that awareness is...and is going along...and, suddenly, you reverse engineer the whole universe and are in charge.

POSTURE TWENTY-TWO
Tolasana (Scale Pose)

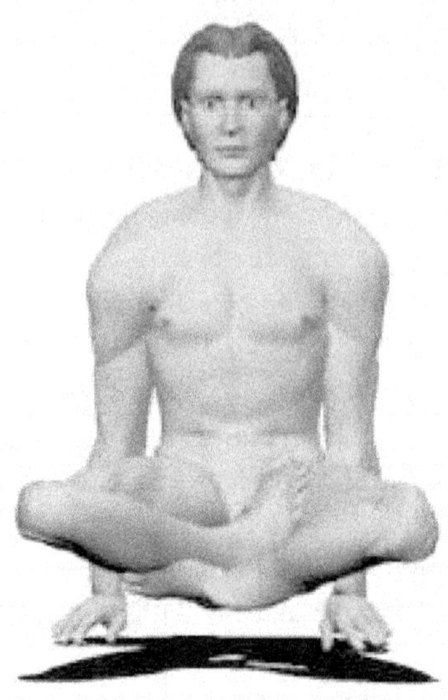

The first of the arm supporting poses. We are going to have to get all the way to a hand stand...plus a few other goodies, if we are going to make it to black belt in yoga.

You can use blocks, if you wish, in the beginning, but eventually you are going to want to just do it.

While the wrists and arms are going to gain much strength, don't underestimate the effects of this pose on the abdomen. You are going to have a core that won't quit.

MORE ON BREATHING

The real Yoga breathing is a matter of cycles.

Assume a pose and breath in for five counts, then breath out for ten counts.

Assume another pose and breath in for five counts, then breath out for ten counts.

You can breath in for 4 or 6 or however many seconds you wish, but whatever the counts when breathing in, double them for breathing out.

Now, something very interesting is going to happen.

First, you will realize that the universe is cyclical in nature.

Second, you will realize that, because the universe has motion (through time), the universe is a wave form.

This will open the door to an appreciation of all waveforms in the universe.

If concepts hold true in the microcosm of the body, they can generally be applied to the macrocosm of the universe.

This is a martial arts concept: what is learned in the small world of the Dojo (training hall, lit.-way place) is applicable in the larger world outside the dojo.

And, you will come to understand that there is a stability in breathing that extends to the things of the universe, and the universe as a whole.

Simply, breathing guides awareness, and as the breath stabilizes, so does the awareness, and you control the universe, so the universe stabilizes.

POSTURE TWENTY-THREE
Bakasana (Crane Pose)

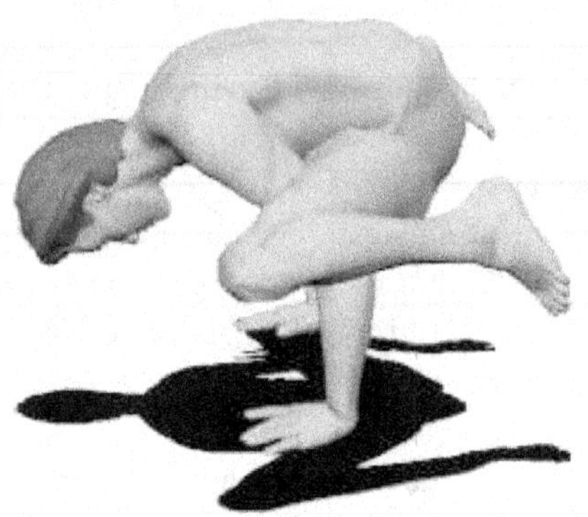

Here is the second arm pose, a little more difficult, but not that big a deal.

Simply place the hands on the floor, place your shins just above your elbows. Voila!

This is a pose of balance. A little strength, a lot of balance. Once you get the balance you'll realize that strength is vastly over rated.

That said, place a pillow on the floor so that your head has some thing to land on when you fall forward.

Believe me, you aren't falling far enough, or with enough speed, to really hurt yourself.

And, you should probably learn how to do a shoulder roll before doing this posture.

Once you no longer need a pillow, spread out a good book and start enjoying yourself.

You are going to get strong wrists, and your abdominal region is going to yell yippee!

UNDERSTANDING REALITY

People can't measure the universe, and they certainly can't make intellectual judgement, if they don't accurately perceive the universe.

Not perceiving the universe, they have false understanding, and so become victim to the universe. Victim of their own creation.

Not perceiving the universe, they create fantasy to replace it. If fantasy, projected from the self, can be trusted over ones own perceptions, one is in deep trouble. (But, don't worry, there is always Yoga!)

Not perceiving the universe, they draw on memories, until memories are out of control and replace ones perceptions of the universe.

Indeed, to the degree that one does not perceive the universe, to that degree one is actually insane. And to the degree that one perceives the universe (directly), to that degree one is sane.

There is a little insane, i.e., political opinions one is willing to change.

There is more insane, i.e. religious opinions one won't change.

There is terribly insane, i.e., a man becomes a serial killer because of what he thinks is going on in this rather sedate universe.

Is there totally insane? Sure. To the degree that one believes the universe exists, to that degree one is totally insane.

Now, doing yoga, sweating, cleanses the organs, and perceptic organs suddenly start to function. And, one finally starts to see reality as it really is. Reality being the projection of the human spirit, it acts as a sort of mirror, and one finally starts to see oneself.

Is Awareness insane? Only to the degree that it cannot be aware of itself.

POSTURE TWENTY-FOUR
Anantasana (Side-Reclining Leg Lift)

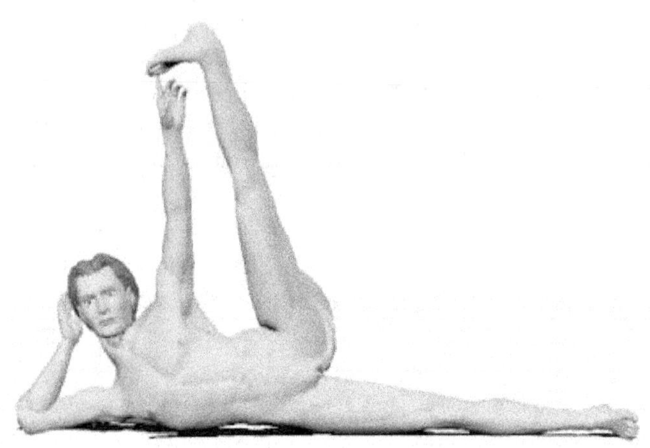

Oh, ouch! You can see my software can't quite get this one. The arm is too short because there is not proper joint articulation at the hip, and the buttock on the upper hip is bulging in a rather unsightly way.

That's okay, as long as you understand that you should be able to hold the foot with your hand, you're fine.

Obviously, this one is going to open up the hips and groin, get those legs in tip top shape.

More important, this is going to set up similar poses, but while standing.

In Yoga, you see, you might strike a pose which is gravity friendly, which is to say it doesn't take much strength, you can focus on your body, and so on.

Then, stand that pose on one foot, and suddenly you have gravity tugging at you. Make everything much more difficult.

That's okay, gravity friendly poses are baby steps, and they lead to the big leagues.

Relax, Breath. Enjoy.

SLEEP

Do you remember The Matrix? Great movie. Very real.

The Matrix existed because when people were used as batteries, there needed to be some place where the being could have existence.

So, in a universe such this one, the spiritual being, once he has accorded the universe power over him, needs a place to go where he can experience his spirituality.

So he sleeps. And, perchance, he dreams.

Interestingly, when I achieved Black Belt I stopped dreaming. Which is to say I stopped having fantasies when I was asleep.

Instead, I started going astral. I would go to places and do things, and it seemed like I...could...almost...take direct control.

Not quite awake, but gaining awareness.

Now, on one level, you need sleep. You need to let the body recharge.

On another level, you need to get out of that body, reaffirm your spirituality, have dreams, know that there is something beside coffin boots and bloody mud and concrete cities and death and taxes and politicians.

There has got to be a hope of spirituality, or...we might just as well fulfill the definition for total insanity.

So, sleep. Have fantasy in dream, and, once progressed in Yoga, or martial arts, or some other discipline, your dreams will become more real, and the real world will become less confining, and you will be more you.

More aware of what your true potential is.

Aware of Aware.

POSTURE TWENTY-FIVE
Setu Bandha Sarvangasana (Bridge Pose)

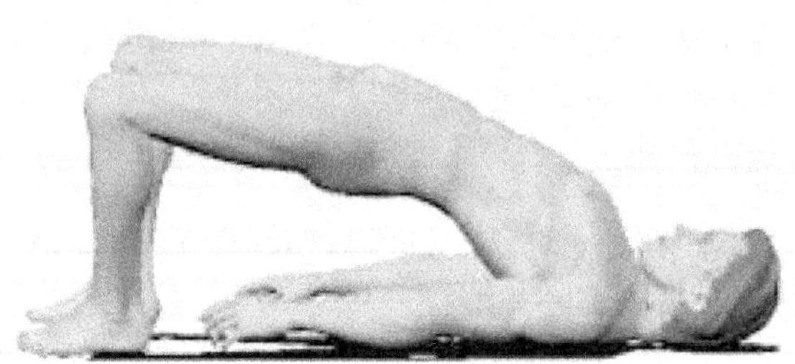

This pose is fantastic for the back, but don't do it if you have neck problems. As always, if you have a specific body problems, use gentler types of poses to edge into the more difficult asanas.

Bridge poses are always wonderful, because they tend to balance all the forward bending motion we do in our normal activities. Thus, if you have pinched nerves, subluxations, and so on, bridging tends to be the cure.

But, be careful. Examine the pose minutely, educate yourself as to how the body actually works.

Stretches the chest and opens up the internal organs. Definitely improves digestion, and relieves anxiety, fatigue, even insomnia!

Here's a fun little move on the right to help you advance your technique!

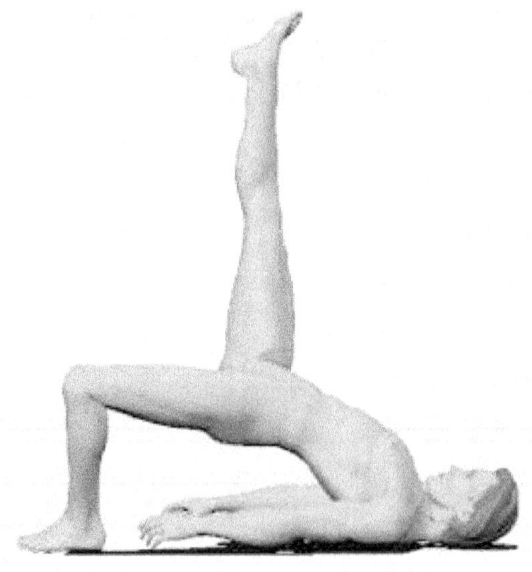

WHAT REALITY IS

Reality is something we made up in order to have existence.

Then we lost control.

The truth of the matter is that in the beginning was the word, and the word was God.

So, in the beginning there was awareness (nothing measurable), and we imagined up all sorts of stuff, and we fixed it in place by giving it names.

Thus, reality continues.

Want to mess with reality?

Simply unname stuff in your head (imagination).

Do it easy enough and stuff actually disappears.

But, to do this, you have to see reality as it is, and that is the hard part.

So unname your wife. When you do this you will drive her insane, and she will want to lock you up.

Which is an interesting reversal of the situation which proves that she creates the universe, and that she is attempting to make something in the universe disappear.

Eventually, she will want a divorce. She will disappear.

Now do this to objects.

People are easy, objects are more difficult to work with. That is because we have fooled ourselves into believing that they are real for so long.

But, listen...an object does not exist, only your name for it exists, and that in imagination.

So the key to controlling the universe is to control the imagination.

POSTURE TWENTY-SIX
Viparita Karani (Legs-Up-the-Wall Pose)

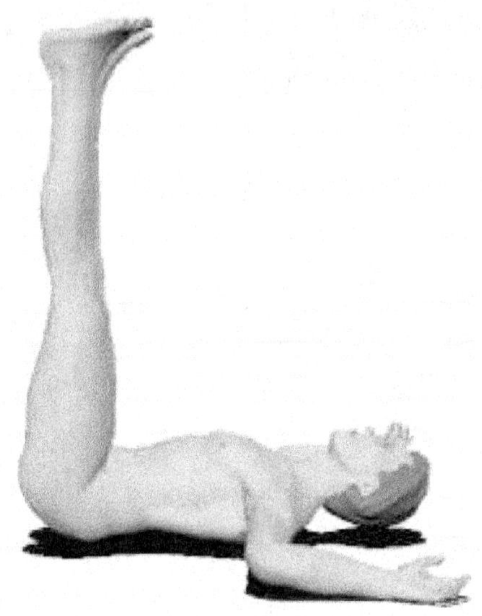

Legs up the wall, ahhh! How relaxing.

I obviously don't have a wall here, but I think you can see what I mean.

Now, when I moved away from the wall I used to use a belt to help me get my legs up and straight. Good for the arms, too.

Once there, I used to advance this pose by moving both legs to one side, then the other. I focused on twisting the torso, but made sure I wasn't overdoing anything.

You know, I don't give extensive instructions, I am more interesting in the Neutronics and the Patanjali and that sort of thing.

Besides, if you just look at your body with awareness, feel where it doesn't feel comfortable, edge very slowly forward with small, subtle motions, telling your muscles to relax and live a little, that's the best instruction I can give you.

CONTROL

If you want to control the universe you must start with yourself.

There is control, and there is chaos...so which would you prefer?
Anything in this world can be gotten through control.
Chaos doesn't get you anything.
So you control the body, which tells the mind to get in control, and thus, you approach spiritual realms, where you exercise ultimate control.
Here is the key: you must exercise your will, and you must not indulge yourself in meaningless activities.
To exercise your will is to want, to desire, to fix your gaze upon an upward path and go there.
To not self indulge is to say no when silly desires come up.
No, I won't drink.
No, I won't drug.
No, I won't prostitute or give in to other pleasures of the flesh.

Yes, I am spirit, and there is nothing else, and I will persist in that belief (read the neutronic scriptures, do the postures, practice the martial arts) until I am awake, and my awareness is aware of being aware.

Simple, eh?
Grin.

POSTURE TWENTY-SEVEN
Dandasana (Staff Pose)

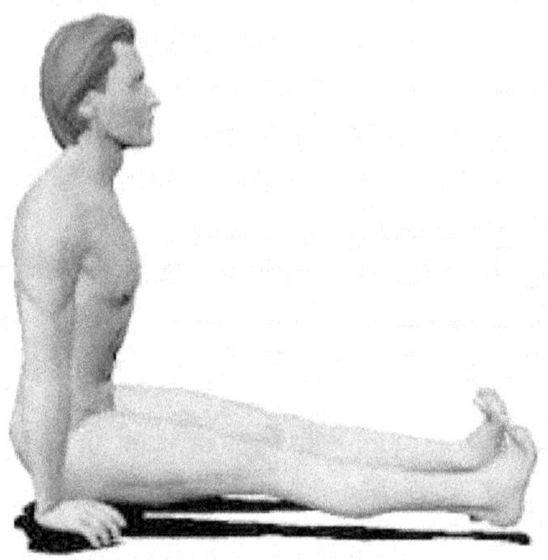

This is the Staff Pose. Very similar to the Legs Up the Wall Pose.

Simply sit, and place the hands upon the ground. You don't have to do much, merely accustom yourself to the right angles at the waist, and the resultant stretches upon the hams.

As I mentioned before, do a pose gravity friendly, then shift your orientation until it is not gravity friendly. You will find all sorts of different muscles and modes of relaxation to work on.

I like doing this with back to the wall, then advancing it by using a belt around the heels. This moves me into folding at the waist.

This pose stretches the back (makes it like 'a staff') and improves the posture.

It tends to help alleviate sciatica.

THE WILL

To see the universe as it is...what a difficult trick.

So you fix your mind on something. An object, a mantra, a...whatever, and you stay fixed.

Your mind wanders.

Refix.

You have problems.

Solve them, and refix.

The world is shaking and quaking.

Refix.

In 1974, when I 'suffered' enlightenment, I realized something.

> For something to be true
> the opposite must also be true.

I was handed the key to the universe. And, I was given something to ponder over for the rest of my life.

From this grew all sorts of martial arts strategies and principles. This became the crux of neutronics, and it enabled me to solve the motor of the universe.

And, it enabled me to solve Yoga.

Mind you, I am not saying it has to be your mantra. But isn't it a bit better than something like 'I want a new car?'

POSTURE TWENTY-EIGHT
Salabhasana (Locust Pose)

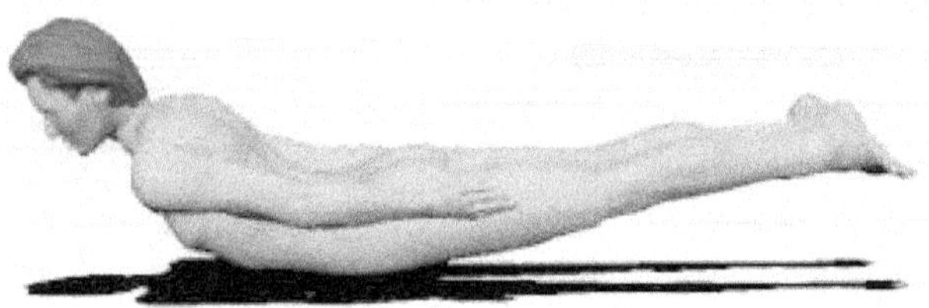

The locust pose, a gentle sort of bridge, which will tighten the back, open the organs, fix sciatica, and generally make one healthy and relaxed.

There is something about the ground (floor) that is wonderful.

We spend so much time looking around, looking up, and we actually hold looking down in disrepute.

But, look down. Relax. Enjoy what is beneath us. It gives us, after all, a firmament upon which to move about and have motion.

GROUNDING

I haven't spoken of grounding, so it is time.

A motor, any motor, needs to be grounded. If it isn't grounded, it will become a universe unto itself and start flopping around.
Loosen the motor mounts on your car engine, if you doubt.
Or, better, loosen that little sideways propeller on the back of a helicopter. Heh.

You ground your body to the earth, and create a motor between planet and body so that you don't fly away into space.

And, on the other hand, you ground yourself, as a spiritual being, to the Greater Awareness.

Sometimes you protest and revolt, even committing vile deeds, but that merely points to the fact that you are protesting something, and thus...are adhered to something.
The Greater Awareness.

The body is grounded, experiences gravity, has sensation, has flow of blood resulting from, and so on.
If there was no gravity, if the motor didn't create some kind of gravity, the motor, and that means all stuff, including the body, would simply dissipate.

The spirit is grounded by being whole unto itself.
The spirit, you see, is a motor of a different sort; it is a universe unto itself.
So when you strike that pose, believe in gravity as it benefits the body, but believe in the uniqueness of your awareness as the true solution to all problems of heaven and earth.

POSTURE TWENTY-NINE
Uttana Shishosana (Extended Puppy Pose)

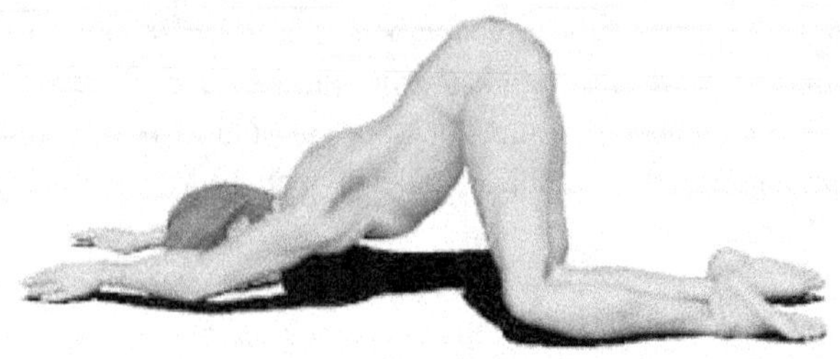

This is a great one for reducing stress. It is like bowing, prostrating oneself, kow towing to the powers that be. And who are the powers that be?

You.

The joy of this pose is that it is like a wave in the spine.

Of course, you won't really find out about waving energy through the body until you get into the martial arts, start doing someTai Chi or Pa Kua.

But, just to hold a pose with a wave in it will go a long way.

THE UNIVERSE IS A WAVE

The whole universe is a wave, you know. A vibration.

If you could make that vibration you could make the whole universe disappear.

Go ahead, study acoustics. Make the vibration, and reverse it, that is, put the crest where the trough is, and the trough where the crest is. The sound will cancel out.

So you could, if could make the sound of the universe, make the universe disappear.

To do that would, of course, require total insanity. Or sanity. One or the other.

Anyway, the sound is supposed to be 'OM.'

And, if you make that sound, on the human level, it is very comforting, the universe aligns with you, and all your dreams come true.

If you make that sound on a body level, then you have realized that you are a spirit and don't need a body.

POSTURE THIRTY
Sphinx Pose

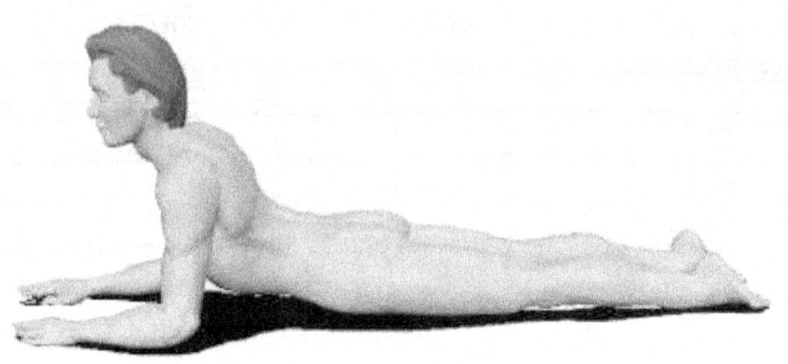

The Sphinx is one of those relaxing restorative poses. You just lay there, propped up and sagging, and the back feels good, and you get regenerated and restored and charged with energy.

Remember, you do the restorative poses at the end of a work out.

Your internal organs are going to wake up, your back is going to stretch, your shoulders are going to get stronger, and all just from restoring yourself to the real you.

Just an interesting note, in Tai Chi Chuan you do the form and you 'store' energy. While this is somewhat different, it is also somewhat the same.

The body doesn't store energy so much as the spirit returns to itself.

Whatever. We like it.

PURPLE BELT

This whole thing of stages and levels and all that is sort of interesting.

You see, if we were in school, we could do grades, but that, as evidenced by todays's school system, is badly abused.

If kids don't get good grades, they change the grading system. One school I heard of, when kids didn't do well, even dropped a class as a requirement. Hmmm.

The real question here is...how do you measure a man?

Not the height and the weight, or the size of the shoe, but the personality, the character, the psychic attributes?

Or, if you really want to get into it...how do you measure virtue?

The best answer I have come up with is...you measure him by his actions.

You measure him by what he does.

Not much of an apprenticeship, but there it is.

Trust them, until they cannot be trusted.

But if they can be trusted, elevate them quickly.

But always watch them.

What? You think this has nothing to do with Yoga?

Au contraire, mon ami.

It has everything to do with Yoga, if you really believe in Yoga.

Yoga is not about sitting in pretzel, it is about learning about yourself so you can change the world and make it into a true reflection of the Greater Awareness.

YOUR THIRD MEDITATION

'I am.'
Simply close your eyes in whatever posture you are in and repeat 'I
am.'

Synchronize it with your breathing patterns.
This is the truth of your universe.
You are The One.

POSTURE THIRTY-ONE
Ardha Uttanasana (Standing Half Forward Bend)

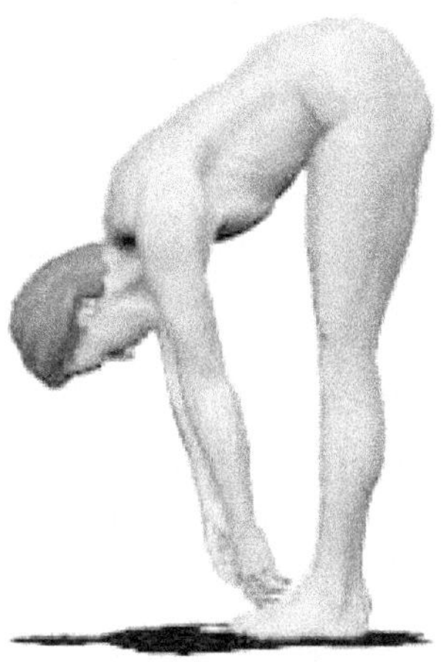

Note: you fold at the waist. You don't stress the back, you fold at the waist.

This is an important stance, as you are going to need to get all the way down to the Big Toe Pose in a short while.

So, don't stress the back, fold at the waist, and relax.

Note: look at your toes, imagine what is under your toes, let the drop happen.

By looking you increase your intention.

This is a funny thing. If you are driving, and you look to the right, the car will veer to the right. The car will follow your intention, even though you have commanded your body to keep the wheel steady and the the car straight.

Intention, you see, rules the world. It is so much more powerful than a simple, fleshy, temporary body.

FORM

The body is a form. A vessel into which you pour life. A vehicle you use to travel around with, while conforming to conditions on earth, while you have body...are imprisoned by body.

In the martial arts form is everything. You learn to control on a vast scale, and on a minute scale, and the lessons translate exactly and directly into the real world of cement and dopes.

In Yoga, form is also everything.

The difference is that in the martial arts the form is on the outside.

In Yoga, the form is on the inside.

This is not an absolute, of course, and quite relative depending on the style of martial art you are choosing.

But, in yoga, instead of motion, you move awareness. You focus on getting rid of body resistance to your intention, and thus your growing awareness.

Now, that all said, there is a Form I do for Yoga, and it is called Yogata, which means...Yoga Kata.

Unfortunately, this form is not available in this book, but rather in the book 'Yogata.'

Good news, it is not expensive.

And, double good news, the Yogata form is a complete holism, covering all potential motions of the body...inside and out.

And, there is plenty of room to expand the form as you become more able.

That is Yogata, and you really should avail yourself and discover the form and expand your viewpoint of Yoga, life, and the Fourfold Path to enlightenment: Scriptural, motion, no motion, and negation.

POSTURE THIRTY-TWO
Dolphin Pose

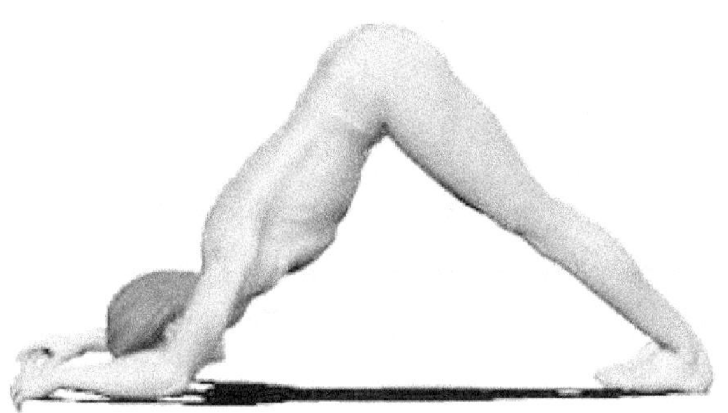

Here is the Downward Facing Dog taken to a more extreme position...The Dolphin Pose.

Same thing, fold at the waist, and keep the feet flat.

You're going to have to really tell the calves and other body parts to relax.

The body is an energy system. Muscles are secondary to energy. So think about geometrical figures of energy, and relax them to happen.

It's not just resistance to muscles, it's resistance to energy.

And, above that, it is the power of the spirit, the I am, to tell the body what to do, and have it do it.

When you can tell the body what to do, and it does it, then you are in charge, and you are well on your way to being aware of yourself as an Awareness.

THE LENSMAN SERIES

We should head back to the Patanjali, but before we do, I wanted to mention one, little thing.

There is a series of books called The Lensmen Series, by a fellow named E. E. Smith.

This series of books details, with great imagination, exactly how imagination works.

It is fiction, space opera, and possibly the most profound novels ever written, and certainly the best and most accurate description of how a human being, a spirit, might imagine energy and make it work.

Reading that series of novels shaped my life at age 15, and excited my imagination to the point where I could figure out how this universe worked, and all the things in it.

POSTURE THIRTY-THREE
Utthita Parsvakonasana (Extended Side Angle Pose)

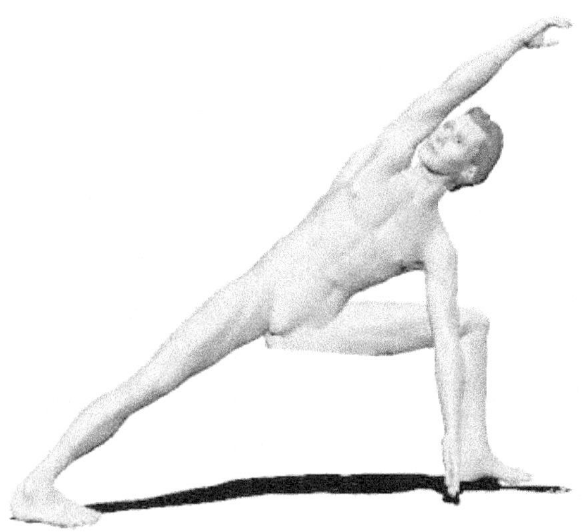

From Warrior Pose you simply lean forward and raise one arm.

Some people wish to go straight up and down with the arms, but I prefer the upper arm aligned with the body.

This is going to stretch the side of the rib cage, which, done both sides, is really going to open up the body and rejuvenate those internal organs. It is also gentle and good for the whole body, from the feet to the fingers, you are going to feel good.

This pose stops constipation, fixes backaches, good for osteoporosis. It stretches and strengthens hips, shoulders, groin, and lots of internal organs.

I don't mention specific organs much, because they are generally all benefited to some degree.

A QUICK SUMMATION

You are a point of awareness.

You create the universe to have being.

You have become victim to the universe.

To return to control of the universe you must grow as awareness.

To return to control of the universe you must cease being distracted.

There is a Fourfold Path (described in this book) which you may follow.

First, you must study sacred (Neutronic) scripture.

Second, you must discipline yourself to be, to awake to your true nature, to be an 'I am.'

Third, you must study motion, that you may handle all the force and flow of the universe, both inside and out.

Fourth, you must refuse to be distracted, you must refuse to fall to the senses, you must hold to yourself an awareness.

Do these things and you will become sacred unto yourself, a universe unto yourself, with all power over the universe.

POSTURE THIRTY-FOUR
Ardha Chandrasana (Half Moon Pose)

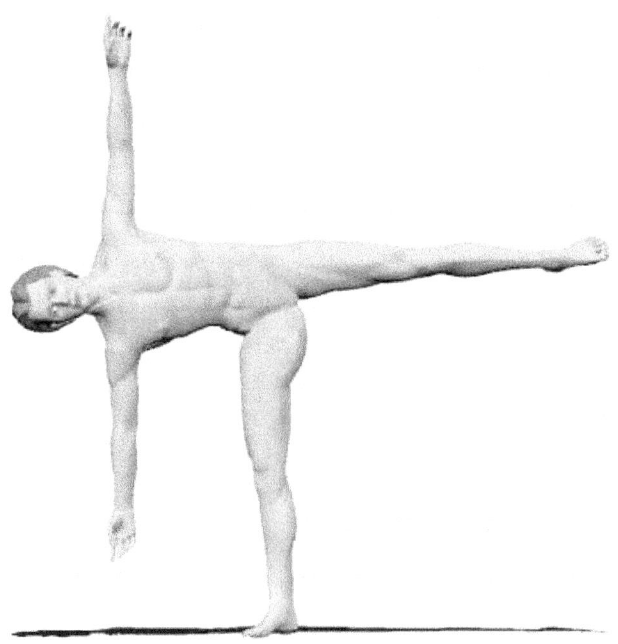

The Half Moon Pose is quite interesting. It requires balance plus.

What is neat is that you can prop yourself up against anything to get into it. The trick is to stay in it after you let go of the prop.

But, having gotten into it, you will be the beneficiary of strong ankles, calves, thighs, knees, hips, and so on. You will also lose anxiety, backaches, sciatica, fatigue, indigestion, and all sorts of other things.

Now, some people say you should touch the ground. Maybe. But I consider that an extra, an expanded version. Cool to go for.

But, it is harder to balance on one foot than a foot and a touch of the finger. So try it both ways, and choose the one that's best for you.

THE OBJECTS OF THE UNIVERSE

Look at an object.

At first, you will be on the outside looking at it.

After a while, you will understand the object from the inside, you will be the object.

Finally, you will realize that the object, no matter how solid it might appear, is an illusion.

It's just a made up thing; a thing of the imagination.

Now, this is the truth of the whole universe; if you can look at an object and realize these things, then that realization applies to every single thing in the universe, and therefore the whole universe.

The whole universe is an illusion. It is something you made up to have existence in.

What? You expect some object to be different from the whole?

Nay. Not so. Tisn't.

So...find an object and start looking.

POSTURE THIRTY-FIVE
Ardha Chandrasana (Half Moon Pose)

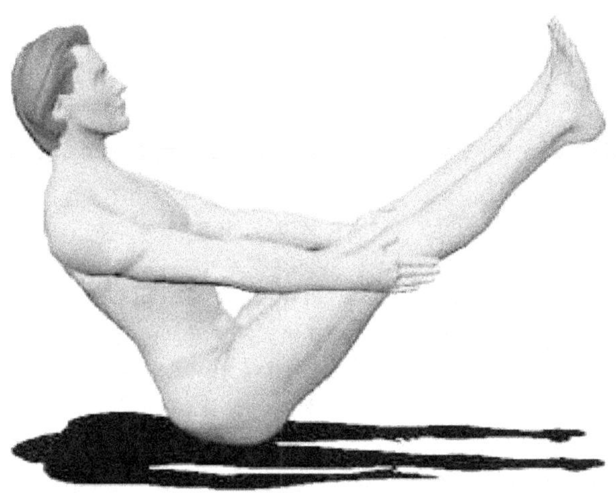

This pose, the Full boat Pose, is going to tuck that tummy and fire up that core!

However, you do have to be careful if you asthma, headaches, low blood pressure, or heart problems. You'll also have improved digestion and lessened stress with this gem.

That all said, the weird thing, this one helps the thyroid gland. Imagine that! This big pose for that little gland. Now, I've never seen the thyroid gland, but I know what the thyroid gland does. That is more than can be said for people who don't pick up a dictionary occasionally...and use it!

THE BODY

The body is a thing. It is an object.

It can be a marvelous and intricate object.

But...just an object.

Now, if you understand that, then you have come to an understanding, and I mean an experiential understanding, of what you are (a point of awareness/ a giver of light/an I am) and what the universe is.

You are aware of the universe as a spiritual manifestation, and that you are in control of it.

Now, very important, you must experience this.

Not talk about it, not read it in books, but experience it.

One of the problems we have gotten into is very learned and scholarly men have written about things they have never experienced. So of what value is their opinion?

In fact, people who have not experienced the truth of this universe usually end up misleading those who would experience it.

There is a reason they haven't experienced it, you see, and this reason stops them from even considering it properly in their writings.

I have experienced it, and you can trust my words, but I wouldn't advise you to.

Question! Look at the words, compare them to other writings, but...make sure you make the distinction between those who have experienced, and those who haven't.

Most of all, develop that gut instinct that tells you whether something is a highway, or...just a small path into the brambles.

I tell you this: a person with no experience wants you to believe. A person with experience wants you to experience.

A scholar wants you to believe what he has written; a person who has experienced himself as an 'I am' wants you to believe you.

POSTURE THIRTY-SIX
Eka Pada Rajakapotasana (One-Legged King Pigeon Pose)

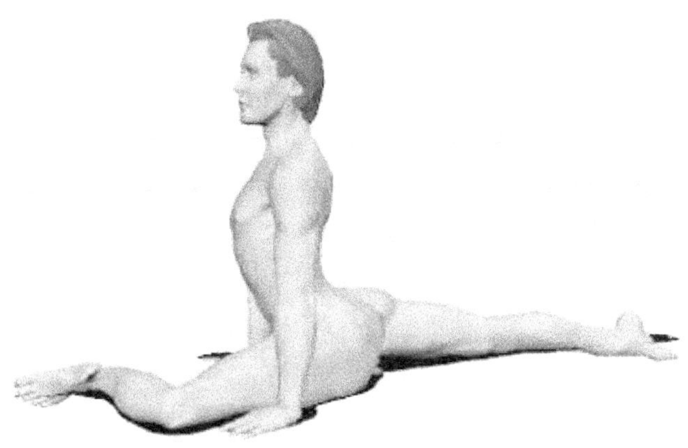

The One Legged King Pigeon Pose is going to open up the groin and the hips big time. It will also stretch the abdomen, and the shoulders.

What's really cool, however, is that it will open the door to advanced poses like the basic Splits (Monkey Pose) and One Legged King Pigeon II, and so on.

However, this is one to avoid if you have suffered from sacroiliac injuries (sciatica), or injuries to the ankle, knee or hips.

It is fun, when in this pose, to stretch it by reaching out to the front, or upwards, or even to the rear.

PUTTING ASIDE THE SIGNIFICANCE OF THE BODY

If you haven't put aside the notion that the body is important, then there are several paths for you.

You can have faith; just keep believing no matter what.

You can seek virtue and do the right thing.

You can be single minded, a fanatic, setting your sights on a goal, and never letting yourself be dissuaded.

Interestingly, these things align with the Fourfold Path of Scripture/ yoga/martial arts/ascetic.

Ask yourself how much of each of these attribute, or properties, that I have listed, are in each of the Fourfold Path.

A monk: consider him in light of keeping faith no matter what, being virtuous and doing the right thing no matter what, being single minded.

A yogi: consider him in light of keeping faith no matter what, being virtuous and doing the right thing no matter what, being single minded.

A martial artist: consider him in light of keeping faith no matter what, being virtuous and doing the right thing no matter what, being single minded.

An ascetic: consider him in light of keeping faith no matter what, being virtuous and doing the right thing no matter what, being single minded.

Do you see the overlap in the paths?

Look, they may not fit together perfectly, but they do fit together. And, it is more important to understand this, than to follow just one path.

It is faster, gives a more expansive view of you and the universe, and, to be honest...it's more fun.

Following the Fourfold Path you are more likely to have a spiritual experience than if you followed just one path.

POSTURE THIRTY-SEVEN
Matsyasana (Fish Pose)

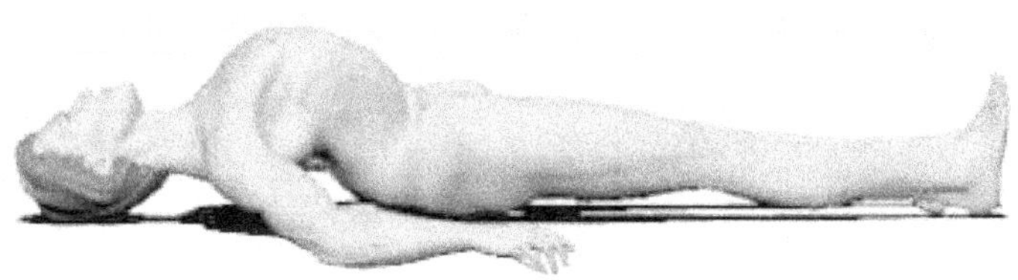

The fish pose thrusts the chest up, tilting the abdomen.

This is a very specific bridge type of pose, aimed at very specific body parts and benefits.

You are going to experience relief from constipation, respiration ailments, backache, anxiety, and more.

However, be careful, find easier poses to work up to this, if you have blood pressure problems, can't sleep, have injuries to the upper spine.

This is a nice one to not spend a lot of time in, but rather just do the up and down motion slowly but gently.

THE FOUR PATHS AND THE MOTOR

When you read scripture, especially Neutronic Scripture, you are seeking understanding. This is like reading an instruction manual before you put something together.

You are trying to understand the whole thing; get the whole picture. This from the viewpoint of the Greater Awareness.

When you are doing Yoga you are seeking to grow Awareness, that you might come to be in control of the motor of Spirit (awareness) and things. Becoming aware of yourself as an Awareness, it is easier to grow that concept to an understanding, and experience, of the Greater Awareness.

When you are doing martial arts you are learning how to handle the universe directly. To be in charge of it. This has much more impact than the other paths. Sometimes it is harder to have a spiritual experience if you are doing martial arts, but the general level of the spiritual being is raised nonetheless, and to a startling degree.

Martial Artists are not confounded by real world problems, and so they can view the real world in a much more honest manner.

There is more to be said, but this is not a book on the martial arts, per se, but more on Yoga, with the added purpose of combining the Fourfold Path.

When you refuse the universe, you are refusing one leg of the motor of the universe, thus going out of agreement with the universe, until you have an experience.

This is a hard path, but the lessons of economy and frugality and such are among the best of lessons.

Think of it this way.

Scripture goes above the motor.

Yoga expands the spiritual terminal of the motor (as opposed to the 'material' terminal.

Martial Arts handles the motor directly.

Asceticism negates the 'real universe' side of the motor.

Take a look at the following picture.

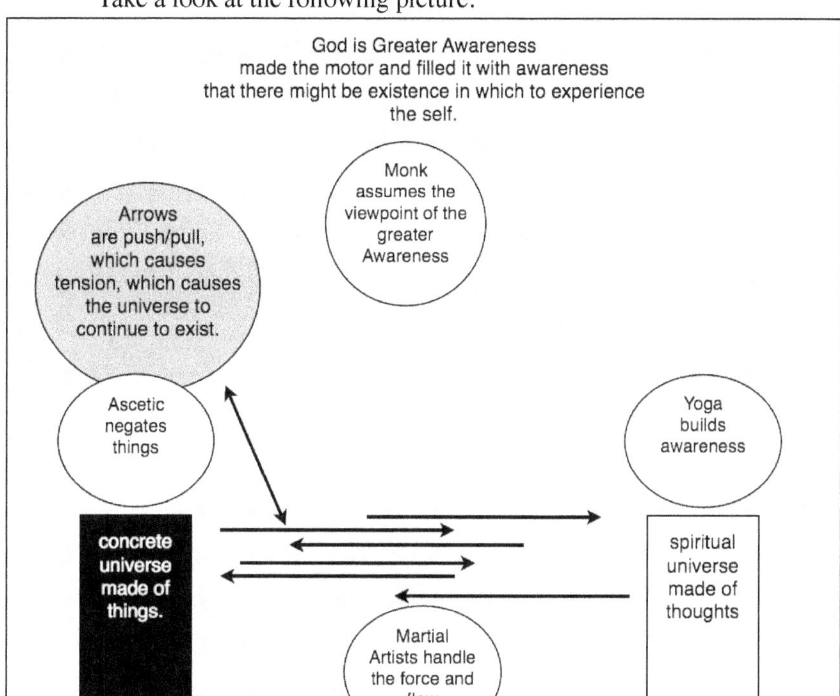

Do you understand how each path of the Fourfold Path attacks the problem of a universe run amuck, insane, and in charge of the spiritual beings who create her?

Do you understand how each of the paths can, if viewed correctly, support the others?

POSTURE THIRTY-EIGHT
Salamba Sarvangasana (Shoulderstand)

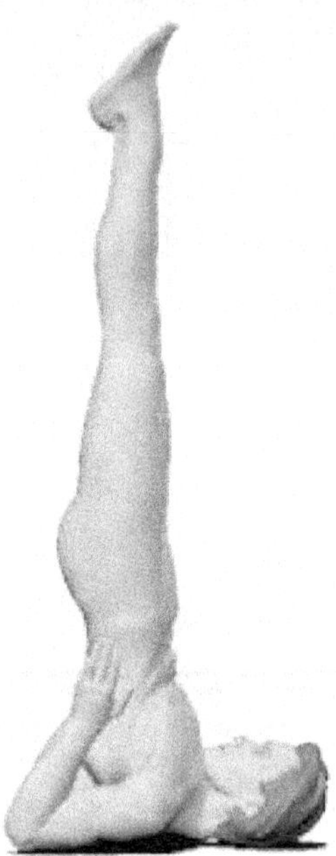

This is the first of the inversion poses. Inversion, in Yoga, refers to upside down. You invert the body. This causes blood to flow downward and nourish the top half of the body. It is also an exercise in balance and orientation of the body to the universe.

The body will, after a short growth period, start to sag. Age. Yikes!

Inversions are excellent for balancing the aging process, and returning you to a fresh, real you. And even in body!

You will struggle for balance, and this will activate muscles on both sides of the various body parts, which will result in stronger muscles on the outside (fast twitch), and stronger muscles on the inside.

THE WILL

People who think of themselves as bodies are weak of will. These are the ones who don't strive to get ahead, are satisfied with a job just because it is 'union guaranteed.'

On the other hand, people who strive to attain a position wherein they are happy doing their work, these people have will.

They have the will to educate themselves.

They have the will to seek out opportunity.

They have the will, and you will find them in a yoga class, or a martial arts school.

They have the will, and you will notice that they are always smiling, always solving problems, always taking the high view of life.

Look, the word will pertains to your desire to succeed, to survive in style, to move to the top, to live a good life by your own wishes.

The unfortunate truth is that society has become a school for the body, and if anyone shows any will they are quickly and immediately discouraged.

My own father became enraged when I said I wanted to study the martial arts. Fortunately, the martial artist who wished to teach me encouraged me, and we always found ways around The Man.

Do you understand how vitally important it is to be unique? To be your own man?

It is the key to EVERYTHING!

POSTURE THIRTY-NINE
Supta Baddha Konasana (Reclining Bound Angle Pose)

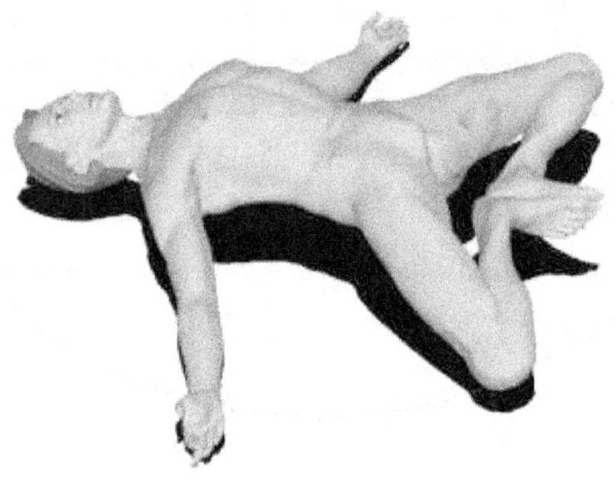

Simply assume the Bound Angle Pose, then lay back into the Reclining Bound Angle Pose.

Puddle into the ground, let the small of the back relax and flatten out.

The hips and groin will open and become loose yet strong beyond belief.

This is a good position for lengthy meditation, but work up to it. It's not a complete restorative pose, but it feels like it, and some people argue that it is.

This pose aids the waterworks. It benefits the prostate, the bladder and the kidneys.

It also helps the heart and improves circulation.

Lot of good things for such a simple pose.

LEARNING

In the Patanjali it says to learn from a master, one who has gone before, and who has freed himself from the toils of life.

However, this society I am in is quite a bit different. I don't know any rich man who teaches Yoga and wants a bunch of apprentices around.

Thus, I feel it far more prudent to advise people to be willing to make mistakes.

You learn a little from succeeding; you learn a lot from mistakes.

In fact, if you make a mistake, are even caught in massive tragedy, start looking around, because inside that tragedy you will find some sort of opportunity, a golden doorway, a portal to an existence higher than the one you experienced before the tragedy.

This is an absolute truth.

POSTURE FORTY
Gomukhasana (Cow Face Pose)

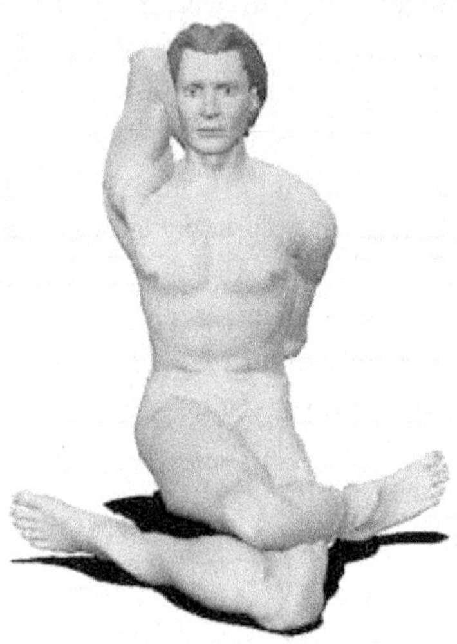

The Cow Face Pose is going to open the shoulders and chest, and strengthen the thighs and hips.

The trick is to get the bones to rest evenly on the rug. There is the problem of the pelvis being slanted, you see. Still, once in, very enjoyable.

Don't you just wonder where the names for the poses come from? One source claimed the knees looked like the lips of a cow, and the arms were the ears. Hmmm. Maybe.

But, what the heck, we don't care what they call it or why, we just want to enjoy and reap the benefits.

WHAT IS A MASTER

This term is loaded in the martial arts, because there are individuals who seek to dominate and conquer and all that sort of silliness.

As if one Aware being could rule another Aware being. That is a joke of the magnitudious first order!

Anyway, a master is somebody who has mastered something. In Yoga, this would be the universe and himself.

This is possible through patience and persistence. The convolution of the poses doesn't matter so much as the depth of the human being.

A fellow who can pick his nose with his elbow is not as worthwhile as a person who helps others sit in the lotus for long periods of time and contemplate, and realize, the nature of the universe, and thus of oneself.

POSTURE FORTY-ONE
Bharadvajasana I (Bharadvaja's Twist)

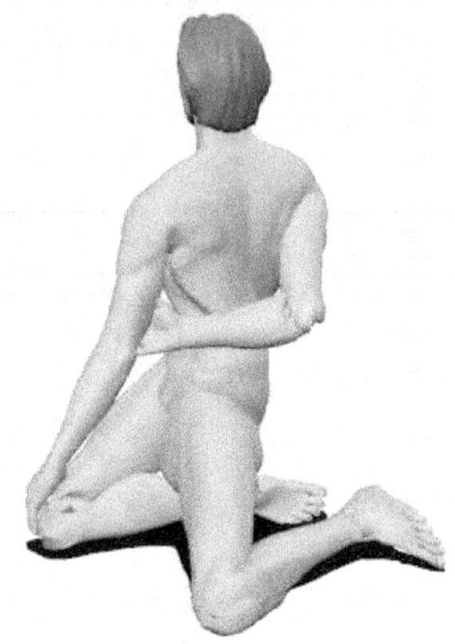

When I have a difficult twist I use a belt in the beginning. Still, many people will be able to get right into this wonderful seated twist.

Bharadvaja was an Arhat, which means 'perfected one.' He is one who has reached nirvana.

Bharadvaja was one of four Arhats asked to remain in the world (not leave the cycle of life and death which binds the unenlightened) to spread Buddhist Law.

Now, there is going to be myth here, and truth. The mix is up to the seeker to define.

What is not myth is the description of the universe in these pages, and of the path available to spiritual seekers.

This pose stretches the hips, spine and shoulders, and it massages the internal organs and relieves stress.

Relax. Breath. Enjoy.

OM

One of the most interesting things to consider is how a spiritual being, one sans body, communicates.

After all, if somebody is, at source, nothing but a point of Awareness…?

The fact is that Awareness, when rubbed up against 'things' causes a reaction. This is 'The Motor,' after all.

So one can effect the real world from the spiritual world simply by increasing Awareness.

It is a sad mark that we have sunk so low that it takes such effort to summon sufficient awareness to move the universe.

All that effort is merely the necessary force to overcome our own reticence to move that which we have created.

Remember, you created the universe, and the only thing that stops you from controlling that universe is…you.

Anyway, an excellent beginning to controlling the universe is OM. It is a sound generated, with or without the body, which embodies intention. Your will. Your desire.

Rub your desire up against something and the world moves.

This is actually not a Yoga thing, it is a martial arts thing. What is called a Kiai, or a 'spirit shout.' The name says it, eh?

In Yoga one attempts to make the OM sound directly.

Don't worry, if you can't figure it out in Yoga, then a few thousand Kiais in the martial arts will do it.

POSTURE FORTY-TWO
Ardha Matsyendrasana (Half Lord of the Fishes Pose)

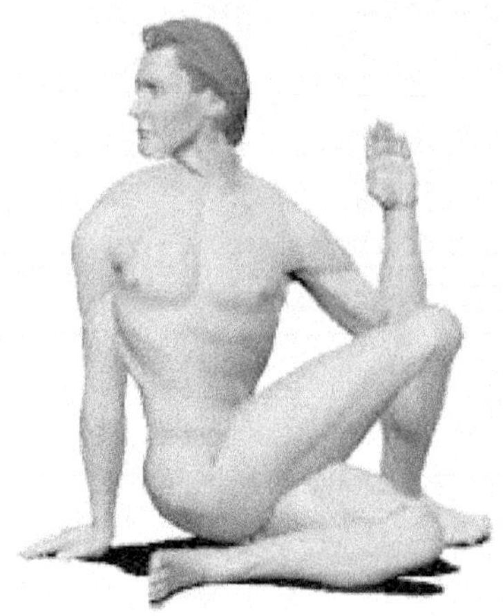

One of those iconic Yoga pose, the Half Lord of the Fishes is a cornerstone twist of the discipline.

This pose works the upper back, benefits sciatica, stimulates the liver and kidney, fills the spine with energy, and all sorts of other things.

If you have had injury to the spine, be very careful. Better to find half twists and do them for a while.

You know, with all seated postures, feel free to avail yourself of a folded blanket or some such aid. Better to ease your way into these things, eh?

ONE SENTENCE TEACHING

A practice I fell into in the martial arts, and one which has provided me with much pleasure and frustration over the years, is called one sentence teaching.

You should, of course, only teach one thing at a time, and you should attempt to embody the central concept of that teaching in a single sentence.

Now, disclaimer, because I am doing more than teaching, I am teaching others to teach, and thus I am frequently guilty of breaking this rule.

But, I advise you to stick to this one sentence discipline, and encourage people to have lengthy discussions as to the exact meaning after class.

One thing that really struck me, when I was learning martial arts, was that if I had a question, the teacher would usually tell me to just to do the form, and the question would be answered. I was astounded, at least in the beginning, when I found this to be a phenomenal truth. Now I take it for gospel, and I always encourage people to do the form to answer their questions.

But, I always ask them after class if they have found their answer, and I give them time for lengthy discussion in the rare event that they have not.

This rule, of One Sentence Teaching, and of letting the asana do the teaching, and not the teacher, works fantastically with Yoga. In fact, it seems it is even more suited for Yoga, where there is little motion and the mind has no recourse but to find its own truth.

The truth of the matter is that the teacher doesn't teach the student, he only provides a space and glow in which the Asana can open the door for the student to teach himself/herself.

POSTURE FORTY-THREE
Virasana (Hero Pose)

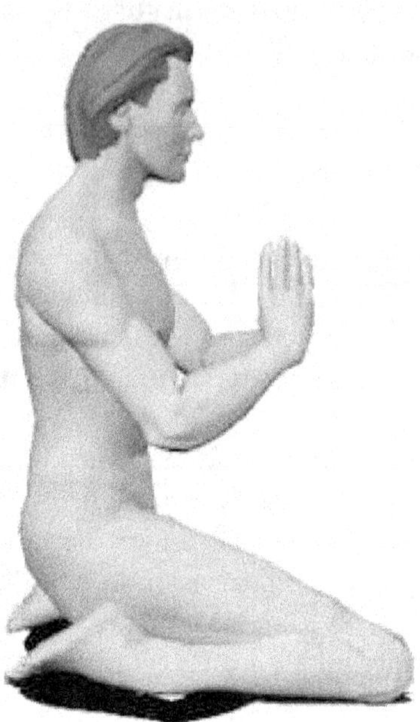

This is the rather famous 'zen' pose, and it is one of the most powerful poses in all the universe.

Of course, one has to go through the pain to the knees, but it is called 'Hero' for a reason, eh? Grin.

Interestingly, this one is good for high blood pressure.

And, I have to say, that though I have presented it with the hands in the prayer position, most people prefer it with the hands folded in the lap.

That's cool. However you want to be a hero is fine with me.

ANIMALS

Want to test your limits? See how well you are doing? Attempt an exercise which will tweak you?

Talk to animals.

It is immense fun to talk to animals.

You don't use your voice, you merely speak to them in images.

You would be surprised at how vocal some animals are, and how well formed their thoughts are.

Indeed, they have well formulated system of ethics.

But it takes, first, creating a silence of mind, and a pointedness of thought.

You see, just as the universe is a motor of two parts, spiritual (light and ethereal) and heavy (walk into a lamp post...ouch!) projecting thought has two parts, and it represents a motor of the mind.

Create silence, project image.

Some people have a natural silence of the mind, and they need to work on projecting thoughts-specific images-into receivers (animals, things, etc.)

Some people have much power of projection, but can't create the silence around it. This is the more common of the two problems people have when it comes to communicating with animals.

But, no matter which area your weakness is, yoga, and martial arts, can help you achieve a balance in this motor of the mind.

POSTURE FORTY-FOUR
Virabhadrasana III (Warrior III Pose)

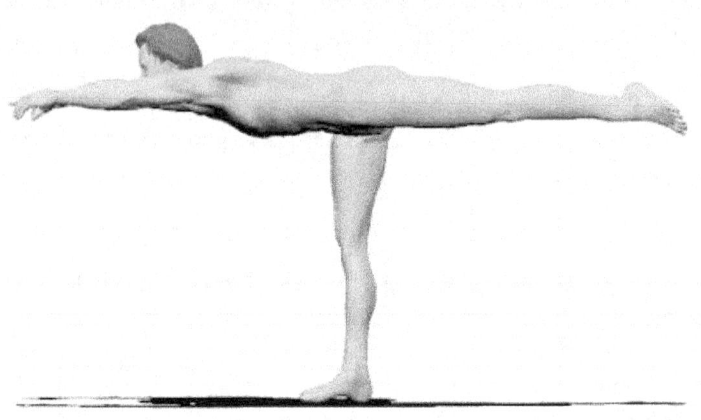

The Warrior III Pose is fantastic for strengthening every body part, either by balance or just strength. Heck, uses every body part, one way or another.

You can get into this by holding on to anything, and then simply let go. Oh, shiver and shake, and...balance.

But, be careful of this one if you have high blood pressure. Use other poses to lower the pressure, then slide into this one.

Now, when you want to step it up, simply strike an earlier warrior pose, 1 or 2, then lean forward at the waist, then raise the back leg.

And, if you want to play a bit, explore different arm positions.

And, if you want to plumb your depths, look at the ground...then close your eyes.

Relax. Breath. Enjoy.

HALF WAY!

We are almost halfway to Black Belt. The next pose will be the official halfway mark.

So, well done!

Halfway there.

Of course, the harder half is coming up.

Quite honestly, I hope you were able to slip through these beginning poses easily, but only if you knew, or had no resistance to, the lessons in this book.

I want to point out something. There are four things happening here: scripture, motionless discipline, motion discipline, and, shall we say...economic teachings?

I know I'm doing a pretty good job, especially as these four disciplines come from different areas, but if you have had any rough spots in understanding, that is the reason.

So, if you went through the beginning postures easily, remember that it is not how fast you go, but how much understanding you accrue, and your study of the postures should bring you to understanding, and that means one thing...you must invest your will, very intensely, in what you do.

To do otherwise is to waste your time.

Fortunately, time is of the universe, so you have plenty of it.

Still, don't dally. Life is worth so much more once you view it from the viewpoint of Awareness, as a spiritual being.

On the next page is the most important posture in all of Yoga, and in the universe.

POSTURE FORTY-FIVE
Padmasana (Lotus Pose)

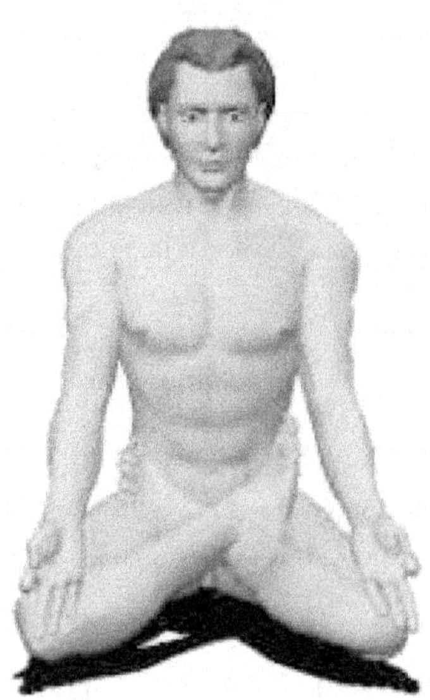

The Lotus. To sit with the back straight, the hands out with the thumb and forefinger circled.

Energy comes, thoughts subside, peace, at last, and the mind sleeps.

But the spiritual being awakes!

This is the pose you should sit and listen in, open up yourself with, explore the universes with.

There is nothing but you, and you is the greatest awareness ever invented in all the histories of all the universes ever.

Forever you.

Ahhh.

BLUE BELT

Halfway up the mountain, but the peak is ahead.

Time to focus your energies, keep your schedule, lean into the wind, and enjoy the race to the top.

At the top, you will find you.

No illusions, nobody whispering in your ear, nothing above you but unlimited sky, and the flowering of the unlimited Greater Awareness of All.

Are you ready?

Good.

Now, go smile into the mirror seven times, and gird thy loins. There is a battle to be unfought.

YOUR FOURTH MEDITATION

The Greater Awareness of All.

Sit in simple pose, such as Easy or Lotus, and consider the fact that you are an 'I am.'

Now, think of a relative that you like, and consider the fact that they are an 'I am.'

Take your time and think pleasant thoughts concerning them.

Now think of a close friend, and consider the fact that they are an 'I am.'

Take your time and think pleasant thoughts concerning them.

Now think of a person you dislike, and consider the fact that they are an 'I am.'

Take your time and think pleasant thoughts concerning them.

Now think of a stranger you passed on the street or during the course of your daily activities, and consider the fact that they are an 'I am.'

Take your time and think pleasant thoughts concerning them.

Now think of a famous person, like a politician or a celebrity, and consider the fact that they are an 'I am.'

Take your time and think pleasant thoughts concerning them.

Think of a person you work with.

Think of a child.

Think of a dead relative.

Think of a dead celebrity.

Think of anybody who comes to mind.

Continue thinking of various people. The longer you do this, the kinder the world will become.

You might find that people will start popping into your mind faster than you can handle them. Force yourself to be calm by listening (Return to the First Meditation, the first meditation is the fix it for all other meditations, should they go astray. Remember, you can listen by looking), and resume the meditation later.

Just because you are causing the world to be 'I am,' and growing the Greater Awareness, and of All, is no reason you should be overwhelmed by their desire to be thought of and including in your magnitudious truth.

If the clamor of people becomes too great, do not do this meditation except occasionally, and, instead, just focus on listening.

You can return to this meditation (it does do the world a world of good) once you have the strength to cease the clamor of the people and listen with a simple thought.

POSTURE FORTY-SIX
Parivrtta Parsvakonasana (Revolved Side Angle Pose)

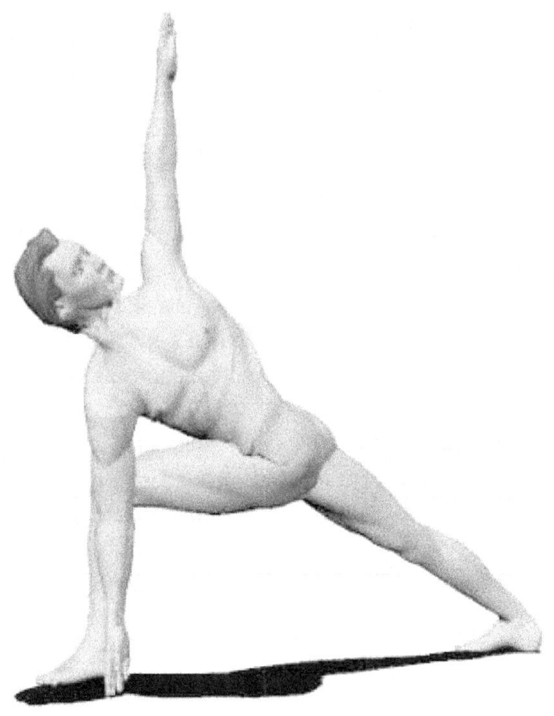

The Revolved Side Angle Pose. Big name, big gain.

The spine is twisted, and the look is forever, and the spiritual being starts to realize how far he can go.

Some people like to Circle the top arm so that it aligns along the ribs and points up the side of the body, one line, from foot to finger and forever. Personally, i like to put the hands in the prayer position.

Keep the rear foot down, and fix up such things as constipation, infertility, sciatica, and so on.

This really is a beautiful pose.

THE MIND

I have said that the mind is a bunch of memories.

Now, you do have mental powers, which seems to attribute more to the mind. But, no.

Mental powers are the psychic powers you have, which includes distractions, and things that you can do, and it is apart from that which we call a mind.

We were talking about silence a few pages ago, so let me use that for my springboard.

To create silence you simply must not allow distractions. Distractions can come from memories (the mind), or one's errant abilities (psychic abilities).

So you can seek out (identify distractions as from different sources, and deal with them accordingly.

The main thing is to be able to create silence.

To be honest, I spent much time pondering over the concept of silence, as Karate means 'empty hands,' and you can't have empty hands without an empty mind.

But it wasn't just my mind that I had to handle, it was the other distractions, and I had a lot of them.

My main weapon was in doing the kata (forms) of martial arts, and learning how to be single minded in my applications.

You should consider being single minded in Yoga, in your life, in your scheduling of life, in everything you do.

Guaranteed, it is the best and surest way, especially when started with a little Yoga, and augmented into full flower with martial arts.

POSTURE FORTY-SEVEN
Lunging

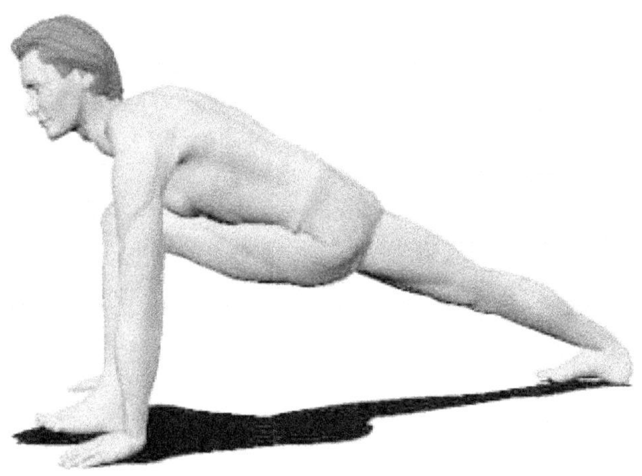

This is very similar to a western 'lunge' in weight lifting and other forms of physical activity.

Regardless, it is a good posture by itself.

It opens up the groin, strengthens the legs, and helps with such problems as sciatica and constipation.

THE DISTRACTIONS

So what causes the distractions? What causes the mind to remember uncontrollably the perception of false realities, fantasies, irrational logic, and so on?

The things that move the spiritual being to untruth are sickness, inertia, light-mindedness, laziness, intemperance, false notions, inability to focus the mind (meditate), or to hold to reality (or a thought) when realized.

If you are sick, get well. Search the doctors until you can find the right help. Read Neutronic scripture. Do what yoga postures or martial arts forms you can until you are able.

Most of all, fix your mind on being healthy of body, mind and spirit, and use all your power to go there.

Inertia is when you are used to acting a certain way, and you let yourself continue, in spite of evidence necessitating change.

You're fat. Stop eating (it's not that simple, but I'll say it anyway, just to encourage you). You're content in a low paying job. Knock that crap off right now! Be discontented, and force yourself to education and unslothful behavior.

Doubt. Don't doubt yourself. You are the strongest, greatest, most wonderful being the universe has ever provided experience for. If you don't believe this, then write the last sentence on a sheet of paper, many sheets of paper, and hang them around the house. Every time you walk through your house and come to the sheet of paper, read it aloud seven times.

That'll do the trick!

Light mindedness. Oh, yes, settle for TV and friends who act cool. Stay buried forever.

Laziness. Get to work. Make a plan. Force yourself out of the sofa and away from the TV. Get going..and i mind now!

Just BTW, the best work outs I ever had in the martial arts were when I didn't want to go, but forced myself to stand up and walk out of the house. Man, I was half out of my body by the time i reached the car, and I ALWAYS learned something profound and wonderful about the martial arts and myself on those occasions.

Intemperance. Nothing wrong with a whiskey once a week, but, durn, do you have to slop the suds every time you get a chance? Don't you realize how stupid you act? Your mental powers are impaired beyond belief, and you aren't much fun to be around. Could you, like, put down the Jim Beam every once in a while?

Slob.

False notions. Marx. Freud. The Council of Nicea. Anything that slants, taints, tweaks, get in the way of you being a perfectly functioning spiritual being.

Unfortunately, modern educational institutions are prime among these corruptions.

Inability to focus the mind. First, make sure your body is healthy. Then, start with the easiest method possible. If necessary, just lay back and listen to music, see if you can stay focused on the lyrics and not let the mind wander.

When you finally realize that you can fix your awareness on the world, hold to it. Don't be distracted. Make up your mind to do what you want to do, and nothing will get in the way.

These are the ways to defeat distraction in this universe.

POSTURE FORTY-EIGHT
Utthita Trikonasana (Extended Triangle Pose)

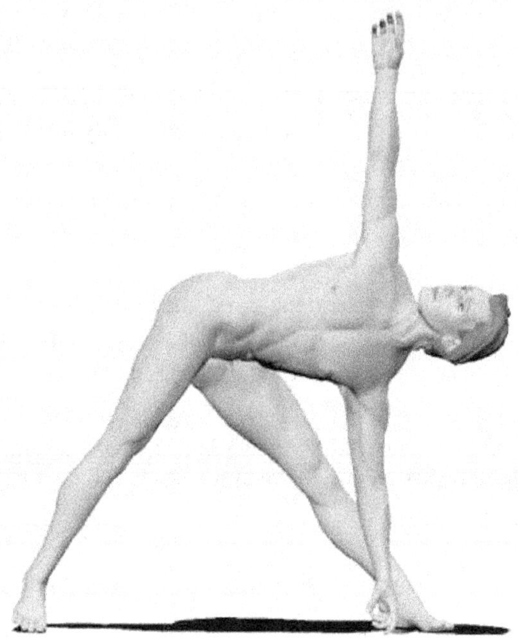

The triangle pose stretches the whole side of the body and, as you do it to the other side, the whole other side of the body. Quite beneficial.

You will stretch and strengthen the sides of the legs and the side of the body, open up the rib cage, massage the internal organs, improve digestion and decrease stress.

Yes, truly beneficial.

Do be careful of this pose if you have low blood pressure.

WASTING WILLPOWER

You are wasting willpower, and the life force of the universe, and your time, if you engage in any of the following activities.

Don't feel sorry for yourself or others. This creates a universe of victims, starting with yourself.

Don't feel sad. This degrades you in all sorts of ways.

Don't not control the body, or mind, or spirit. To not control is to breed chaos.

Don't waste energy. Learn how to be economical and frugal.

I don't usually like to give out 'don'ts,' it is much more pleasurable to provide rules and regulations in a positive manner that people can take them positively and with a smile.

But, the nature of these offenses, and they are offenses...offenses against you and the universe you create...are such that I felt the need to go a bit bleak.

If you have any trouble understanding this data, or adhering to correct principles in your living, you should probably avail yourself of 'The 24 Neutronic Principles.' (ChurchofMartialArts.com)

POSTURE FORTY-NINE
Bhujangasana (Cobra Pose)

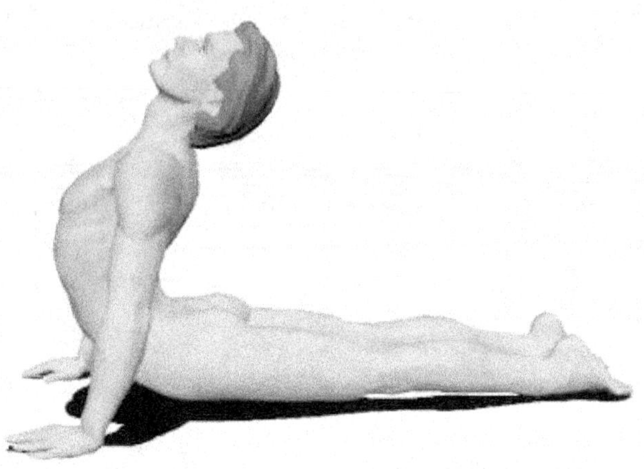

Similar to the Dog Faces up Pose, the Cobra Pose is more of a back bend. Thus, do the Dog, and learn to bend over backwards in your efforts. Nice, eh? Grin.

Make sure you press the hips and waist to the floor on this one.

You will enjoy a stronger spine, firmer buttocks.

You will also stretch the chest and open the heart and lungs, and wake up those abdominal organs.

This won't be a good one to do if you have a headache.

Be aware that your body heat may increase, and you may experience sensations of energy from the Kundalini (power coiled at the base of the spine).

Don't try to force heat or energy, simply relax, do the pose, and get out of the way of your inherent abilities.

ENERGY

Energy is the capacity for work. Interesting, eh? You thought it was some invisible sort of something that...no, it is merely the capacity for work.

Now, life force, chi, prana, whatever you want to call it, is different.

Want to measure your prana? How awake are you physically?

If you need lots of naps, have trouble focusing, you may be weak in Prana.

But, doing the poses, and then, especially the martial arts, you will find that you are able to tap in on a totally unlimited supply of life force energy.

The capacity for work will be almost silly once you have energized yourself through posture and motion.

Now, a little treat. Want to stay awake late at night? Maybe you're pulling a shift and you don't want to be acting tired?

Count fast.

That's all.

Count fast.

Aloud is best, but even silent is of benefit.

Count fast, and everything starts to speed up.

Heh. After a while you're going to be wondering if counting slow will slow you down a bit. I mean, you're going to think it is unnatural, and be afraid you won't be able to sleep in the morning.

No, counting slow won't put you to sleep.

And, don't worry. You won't have any trouble sleeping once you hit the sheets.

POSTURE FIFTY
Halasana (Plow Pose)

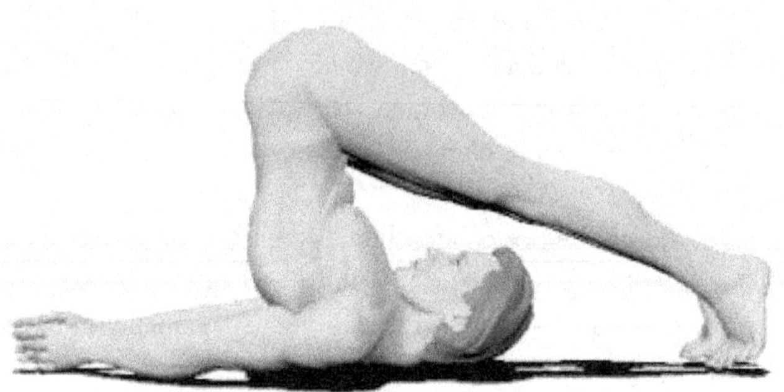

This pose is fun, once you get all the way over and connect your feet with the earth. Just don't forget to clasp your hands. Heh.

Obviously, this one is going to stretch the spine, and massage those internal organs, and even help out old Mr. Thyroid.

Mr. Thyroid determines rate of growth, and that means...how fast you grow old.

Interesting, eh?

And, you get rid of headaches, backaches, insomnia, infertility, and a few other things.

But, don't do it if you've got diarrhea, or neck injuries.

Relax. Breath. Enjoy

HOW TO MAKE THE WORLD WAKE UP AND BE HAPPY!

You know, life can be so easy.

Be happy, and associate with happy people.

Don't mess with sad people.

Fix your attention on goals, don't waver, and enjoy the steadiness of Awareness that accumulates.

Get rid of self-indulgence; just say no. And loudly.

Refuse fantasies and deal with the real world.

The thing is this...you create your own world. You have choice as to the people you hang out with, and the things that you do.

And the fastest, best, easiest way to make your world wake up and have fun is to...make people happy.

No, don't be a comedian (unless appropriate)!

But, help others enjoy their lives. Provide jobs for willing workers, and help them better themselves so they aren't tethered to you forever. Be charitable to those in need, if they really are in need.

Discover those who are duplicitous in their efforts, and no matter how much you like them, even love them, encourage them to their own path, and keep their path separate from yours.

Boy, is this hard, especially when it is a family member that is being less than spiritual.

But, there it is.

POSTURE FIFTY-ONE
Sasangasana (Plow Pose)

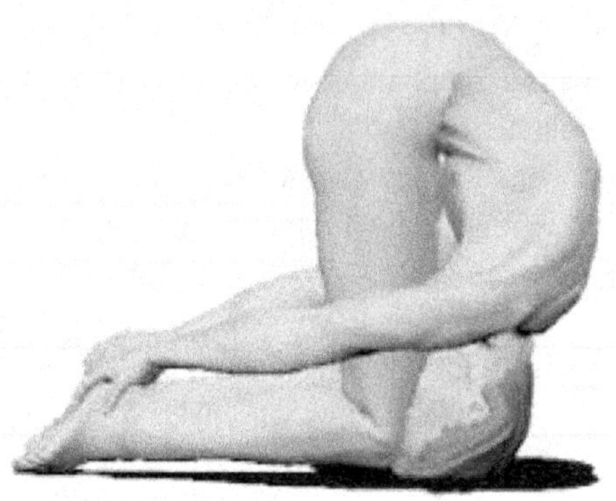

Here's the Rabbit Pose. Simply kneel, bend all the way over and place your head on the mat and grab your heels.

It's a tidy, little pose, very restful, but make sure you don't try it if you have had neck or back injuries.

Best to go into this one from the Child's Pose.

Will help digestion and relieve any abdominal difficulties.

VIBRATION AS A CURE FOR DICHOTOMY

The universe is dichotomous, everything in the universe is dichotomous, which is to say, two terminals make a motor in everything.

Two halves to the body, a top and a bottom to a tree, cells have two terminals (elements), and even the lowly atom has a proton and an electron.

That is where Neutronics comes from, incidentally, the neutron does nothing, has no mass, has no charge, positive or negative, it just sits there and the proton and electron play for it.

That said, when something is out of tune, that means the balance is not right, and one of the terminals is doing all the work, and the other not enough.

To fix this we need merely to understand vibration.

Do a backbend, feel the extremes.

Then do a forward bend, feel the extremes.

Alternate.

Do you understand what we are doing?

We are moving back and forth, like a guitar string, and the string, or the body in this case, will go back and forth, and when you stop it will have found a balance.

And, balanced, the body will be able to cure itself.

Of course, you have to explore all the potentials of posture, and the opposites for these potentials, to insure that you vibrate the body in all its particulars.

POSTURE FIFTY-TWO
Supta Virasana (Reclining Hero Pose)

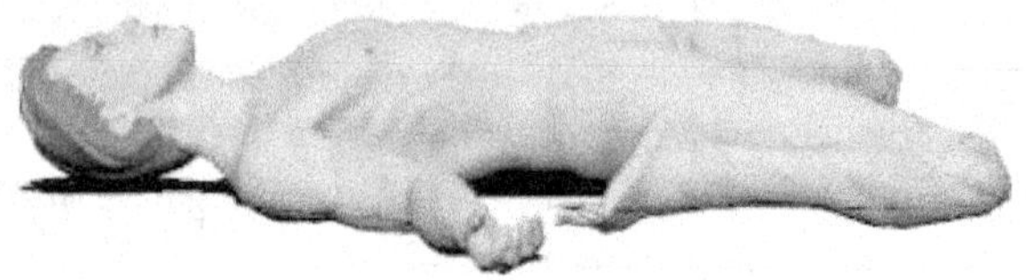

Sit in the Zen position (Hero's Pose), then simply lean back until you are supine upon the floor.

Take your time, let the small of the back flatten out and puddle into the ground.

The heels should be up against the side of the buttocks.

Now, this pose is going to stretch the stomach and thighs, but it is going to do a lot more, too.

Arthritis, Infertility, high blood pressure, insomnia,diarrhea,respiratory problems, sciatica...even varicose veins and flat feet, are going to be helped by this posture.

So, take your time, focus on relaxing each, individual body part that gets rigid, and let yourself go.

THE GEOMETRY OF SPACE

One thing that has aided me greatly is the visualization of geometric shapes in space.

In the martial arts I would examine my forms to see was I standing with the legs a box, a triangle, some combination of the two?

Did my arms configure as circular, where were the joints, was there a free flow of energy through the geometric shapes?

Are the legs a torus through which energy flowed? Which way did the energy flow? Was this effect by breathing and dropping my weight? (The answer to this last was yes.)

And, more motion happening in the martial arts, what was the weave and warp of energy as I went from one stance to another, from one technique to another.

This visualization encouraged me as a martial artist, and gave me incredible benefit. And, remember when I mentioned The Lensmen Series? This visualization of geometry in space was the idea I came up with (amongst others, many others) because of reading that series of books.

If you want a full description of geometry in space, and how the Aware Spiritual Being used that geometry to create the universe, you need to read some of my works on Neutronics. (ChurchofMartialArts.com)

POSTURE FIFTY-THREE
Dhanurasana (Bow Pose)

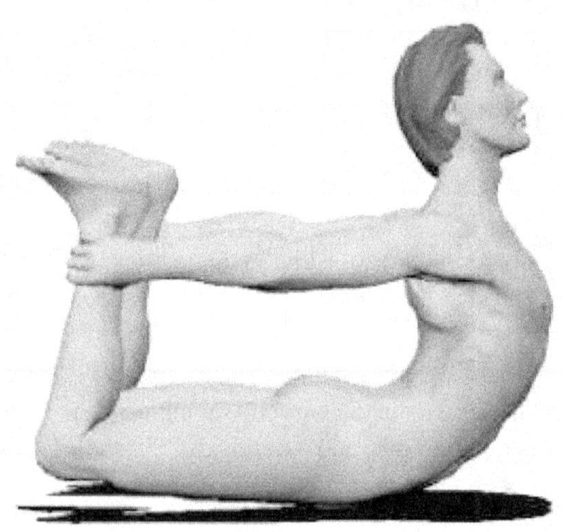

This pose, the Bow Pose (after an archery bow), will stretch your thighs, groin, belly, back, legs...everything.

And, it will help constipation, fatigue, anxiety, respiration, and all sorts of other things.

However, avoid (work up to) if you have headaches, blood pressure problems, insomnia.

Remember, your thighs should be slightly lifted.

And, if you have trouble breathing, just relax, try to breath into the back of your lungs, and persist.

The thing that is nice about this pose is that you can hold your ankles and really relax.

A few times and you will be an old hand.

A MATTER OF PERSPECTIVE

The monk reads scriptures seeking the divine word of God.

The monk holds a posture while attempting to fathom the Greater Awareness, that he might understand himself as a lesser version of the Greater Awareness.

The yogi holds posture seeking the Greater Awareness.

The yogi emulates the greater universe that he might join his lesser universe with it.

The martial artist handles the force and flow of the universe, that he might understand the divine inspiration that moves all.

The ascetic refuses the universe.

The ascetic refuses the universe that he might find its opposite, his own Awareness.

Do you see how these seekers touch upon each others paths?

Do you see how the knowledge of one of the Fourfold Paths might encourage and benefit the knowledge of one of the other of the Fourfold Paths?

It is a matter of perspective.

If you think there is only one path, then you are refusing information and experiences that might open up your progress.

If you study all paths, you may still hold to one, but you will have greater perspective, and thus be able to travel ever faster.

And, the body dies, so you must hurry.

Do not waste time, do not waste energy, else you have to do it all over again.

Yes, lifetime after lifetime you can accumulate knowledge, but who is to say that you will have such clean path as is before you in these pages?

Who is to say that you will not be set upon by the wild animals of this universe, the unaware spiritual beings, who wish to derail you just to protect themselves from their own lack of spiritual essence?

Who is to say that the gains of spirituality you make this lifetime won't be erased next lifetime? Your condition actually made worse?

Why do you think this universe has lasted so long?

Why do you think you have had to live lifetime after lifetime for so long?

The idea that you can dilly dally and take your time has caused you more misery than you can imagine...in your temporary, little body.

POSTURE FIFTY-FOUR
Marichyasana III (Marichi's Pose)

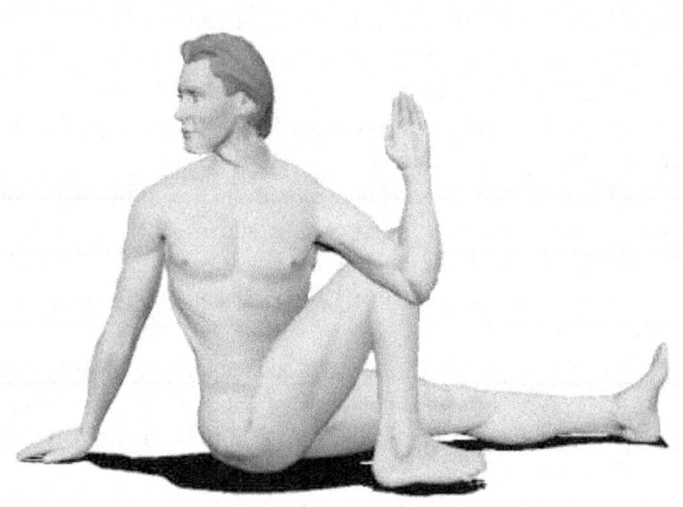

Marichi means, loosely, light from the moon. He's the son of Brahma, and one of the seven gods who oversee Dharmic Law. Good job, if you can handle it.

In this pose you will stretch and twist at the same time, which will help the spine and lower back immensely.

By by to asthma, digestive disorders, sciatica, and all sorts of other things.

Once you pass the half way mark in this book, achieve the level of Blue Belt, the poses are tougher, but they bite more. You are going to experience more benefit in a greater variety of ways.

The main thing, however, is that you will become sharper in intellect, more Aware.

Remember, you are only using the body as a via to improve the focus of intellect that you might be more aware.

BTW, Marichi's Pose is sometimes referred to as the Sage's Pose.

BREATHING

Here we are at breathing again.

Please remember, I am not being redundant, merely taking you to deeper levels.

Breathing, the old in and out, is a vibration, is it not?

Thus, by breathing deep, and controlling the breathing through posture, you not only become sharper of intellect and more aware, you vibrate the body on the cellular level.

Oxygen passes in and out, causing all the cells to vibrate, to cycle through their existence, to occur in complete vibration.

Breathing, it is the life force incarnate. It moves the body, vibrates the body, causes the body to wave through existence, and on many levels.

Go on, try and do without breathing for a while. You'll find out. Heh.

POSTURE FIFTY-FIVE
Janu Sirsasana (Head-to-Knee Forward Bend)

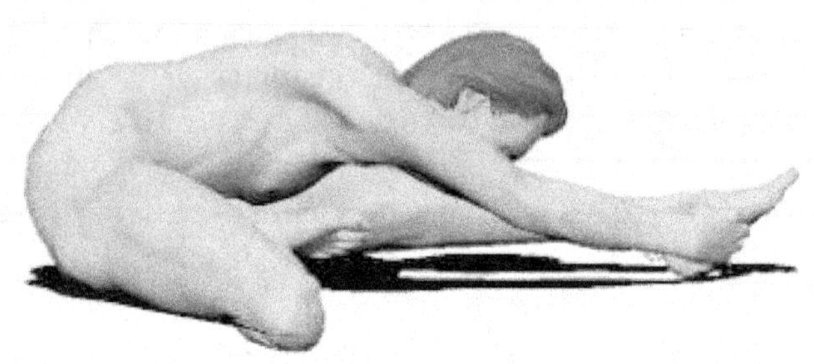

A great bend and stretch. From a bound angle simple extend one leg and bend, or, stretch one leg, and pull the other foot into the thigh.

Aside from the basic three dimensions, X, Y, and Z, you've probably figured out that all you have to do in Yoga is bend, stretch, and twist.

What you should do is figure out the percentages of each. Guaranteed, this odd bit of knowledge will help you.

Anyway, the Head to Knee Forward Bend is going to deal with depression and relieve anxiety.

Isn't it interesting how manipulating the body, learning that you can control your body, leads you to control of deeper levels of your spiritual being?

This pose also helps the live and kidneys, high blood pressure, sinusitis, and lots of other goodies.

One thing you might do, if you wish to be enterprising and leap to the head of the class, is divide the poses up into categories: bends, stretches, twists, and see which categories tend to fix up which ailments.

It's a very interesting study with some very interesting results.

EATING

I'm probably going to get back into the Patanjali again, but before I do I wanted to mention diet.

There are so many diets these days, everybody has an opinion, and most of the stuff you read is junk.

There are diets based on blood type, the zodiac, body shape, and so on and so on and....

Look. I know what I am saying is going to upset lots of people, everybody believes in macro or vegan or whatever, but I haven't seen many diets based on science.

What, exactly, does the human body need?

And, what are the factors that change those needs from individual to individual?

The problem is that nobody has matrixed the human body and figured out all of the systems, how they intertwine, and what each needs to get balanced and stay balanced.

So, the solution is for you to do it for yourself.

Start investigating the science of nutrition, not the fads, and figure out what your body needs and wants.

And everybody is going to be different.

As for myself, without going scientific on you, I base my diet on the following factors.

Main factor number one: the caveman diet. If I can't pick it or kill it, I don't eat it.

What this means is no synthetics. Honestly, the body doesn't like synthetics, even something as simple as flour.

I find that my body gets lean and mean, with no cravings, when I eat caveman.

Main factor number two: most of the vegetables these days, most of anything you'll find in the grocery stores, has been preserved, dyed, made salty or sugary, msg-ed, and so on and so on, and...the big one, modified right down to the DNA.

Modified like in radiation or the DNA actually altered through chemical and biological processes.

Look, if you eat a watermelon, and the seeds are gone, what is that going to do to your seed?

If you eat a cow that has been made fat by hormones, what is that going to do to your body?

Main Fact number three is a constant mix and blend of everything I hear as I search for what is uniquely right for me. For instance, I take into effect items like the ones mentioned in the next few paragraphs.

The human body was developed over thousands of years with a dependence on Barley. Interestingly, when I eat barley I feel very different. Not energized so much as deeply stable, like somebody just pulled the fulcrum out from under my teeter totter.

I was raised on a basic diet of meat, starches, and vegetables.

I crave certain sugars, but when I eat meat, the craving is reduced to gone.

Red meat makes me loggy.

And so on.

POSTURE FIFTY-SIX
Parivrtta Janu Sirsasana (Revolved Head-to-Knee Pose)

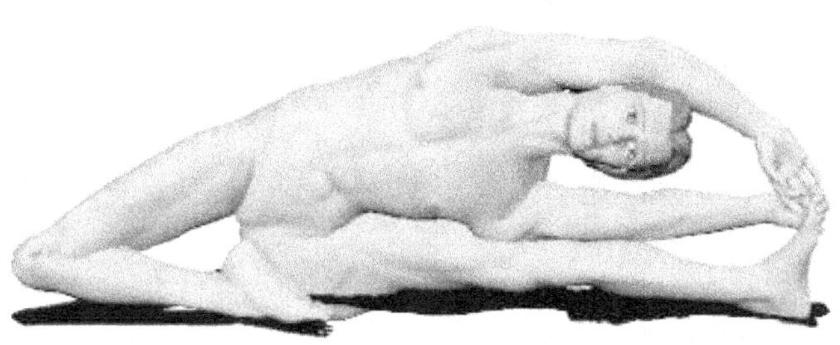

This is the same as a head to knee forward bend, but to the side. My software couldn't quite get the hips down, but it did a fair job. You simply stretch one leg to the side, and fold, as in bound angle, the other foot. Then you stretch over the top and open up the rib cage, shoulders, groin, spine, and the whole side of your body.

Your digestion is going to improve greatly, and your kidneys and liver are going to be jumping for joy.

Don't you just love being healthy?

Don't you just love the spiritual glow that is starting to emit from your body?

A nice variation is to reach with the lower hand to the back foot. Very Beautiful.

OH, AND ONE LAST THING...

One last thing before we return to the Patanjali...at this point you should be looking around for a yoga teacher.

Now, to be honest, my first yoga teacher was a simple CD. Ten bucks on Amazon. And, it was great stuff. Nothing too difficult, but it moved me on.

Then I downloaded an app. Sheer joy. Multiple layers, I could tailor my work outs.

And so on.

But...at a certain point you should seek out professional instruction.

As the poses get more difficult, you are going to need tips and hints about how to get from one pose to another, how to take advantage of blankets and straps and blocks and things so as to better ease into the game.

You have educated yourself with this book, so you should be able to avoid the quacks or the people who talk a good game.

And, if you're a smart fellow or gal-and by that I mean you have common sense-you can continue with just this book. Heck, if you read this book, study some anatomy charts, have a fair idea of what is really going on with your body with some of these asanas, then go for it.

I had the benefit of decades of martial arts. I had looked at the charts and analyzed the motion of muscles and bones and how they worked together, nerves and nerve clusters in connection with Dim Mak (poison hand death touch), and all sorts of things to do with the spine and the connections within the human body, so I was fair educated

But most people don't have that. So, think about it. Maybe go down ask if you can watch a class, talk to the yogi afterwards, and see what you can see.

POSTURE FIFTY-SEVEN
Paschimottanasana (Seated Forward Bend)

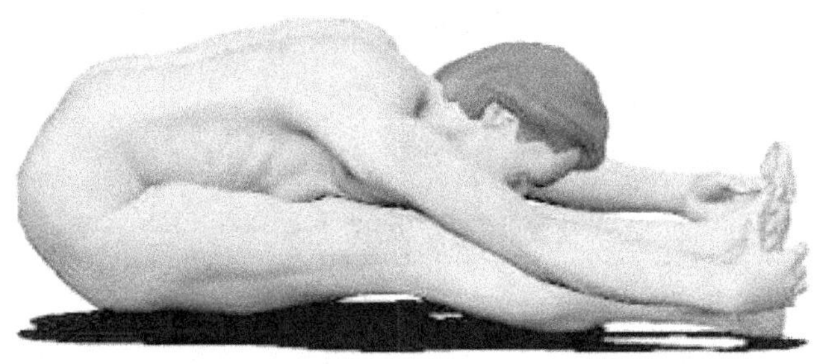

All righty! A good, deep bend.
Remember to fold at the waist.
Once you get those feet, hold on, and relax the rest of the body.

No twist here, just stretch the hams, spine, and shoulders.
You'll do without stress and depression and anxiety. Now that's a great triple whammy.
Your kidney and liver are going to celebrate, and you're going to be rid of fatigue, get a little extra appetite, and generally feel like dancing all night.
And why not? Eh?

LET'S TALK ABOUT THE UNIVERSE

I have said that you are a spiritual being, and that you create the universe, and this is true. You, the Awareness, project the universe. You are like a movie projector, and the universe is like a movie.

Now, something you should remember, when you can finally still the mind, eliminate distraction, you are going to feel like you are the universe.

This is often mistaken for the 'joining' that is Yoga.

And, it is a good thing to experience, but don't you dare stop on that.

Don't stop until you twitch your toes and it rains, until you crook your finger and crowds gather to celebrate their goodness, until you have a thought...and it manifests.

It's not enough to think you are the universe, you must go beyond that and make the universe work.

You must operate the universe like you would drive a car.

One heck of a car, eh?

Grin.

POSTURE FIFTY-EIGHT
Anjaneyasana (Low Lunge)

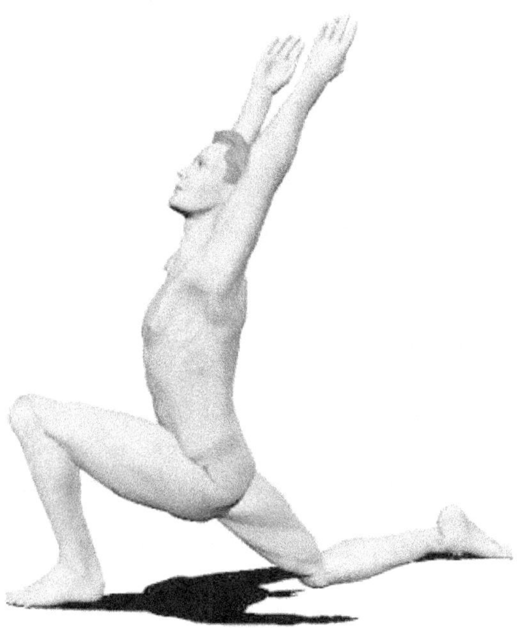

The Low Lunge. Stretch the rear foot a bit further back, just enough to make a softer curve of the back knee.

Stretch the spine and shoulders, open the hips and groin.

Good for deep leg strength, and will even improve the sacroiliac connection.

You can hold this one a while, doing the half count breathing in, and the double count breathing out.

While you can just step out and lunge, it sometimes looks a bit clunky. You might want to sink from the high lunge, or perhaps, just for kicks, swing up from the dog faces up.

IMMORTALITY

The goal is to accumulate enough awareness, to lose enough resistance to the idea of yourself, that you live beyond your body.

The body dies, but that which is you, the spiritual being, the awareness, goes on.

We are trapped in a cycle of dying bodies because we are dwindled in awareness. If we become more aware, we will remain aware after the death of the body.

Examine literature. The gods were immortal. That just means they were aware enough that they could break out of the cycle of going and getting new bodies.

So, do you want to be a god? All you have to do is accumulate enough awareness, lose enough distractions, not be trapped by all the motors that you have created.

When you die, break the motors, give up the motors for awareness.

Do you understand?

POSTURE FIFTY-NINE
Parivrtta Trikonasana (Revolved Triangle Pose)

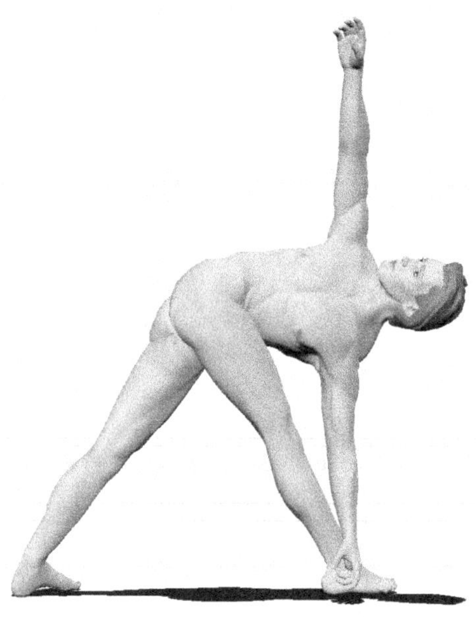

The Revolved Triangle Pose is one of those fun ones. You can build a quick routine that is funtastic.

Stand up with the legs spread.

Fold sideways at the waist to a triangle.

Revolve (twist) to a revolved triangle.

Reverse to the beginning, then do the other side.

It's just downright fun.

And, you can play with different arm positions, and even with dipping into a warrior stance.

This asana works the spine, fixes up digestive probs (well, duh, look at the twist in the belly, that's going to grind up anything you put down there), and even fix asthma!

THE JOY OF SELF

When one actually perceives the universe as it is, a profound happiness wells as if from inside.

When you can still the distractions, control the body, mind and spirit, then a calm will wash over you.

This inner peace, this glow, is such that it cannot be described by pen and paper.

It is like the satisfaction after a long days work, but tenfold. A hundredfold.

Now, the way it happens is like this: one studies and disciplines oneself, and becomes better able to handle the force and flow of the universe.

And, one becomes more aware of the self as an aware being.

Awareness increases, and distractions decrease, and, finally, one starts to come into that unique, spiritual glow that is oneself.

And, one joins to the universe, which is to say, they think they are the universe, and the inner glow turns on full force.

That is what is going to happen...if you make it happen.

But you must make up your mind not to be distracted, not to be turned aside, neither from your own delusions, nor from non-spiritual beings.

You must dedicate yourself over and above the things of the universe.

POSTURE SIXTY
Ardha Bhekasana (Half Frog Pose)

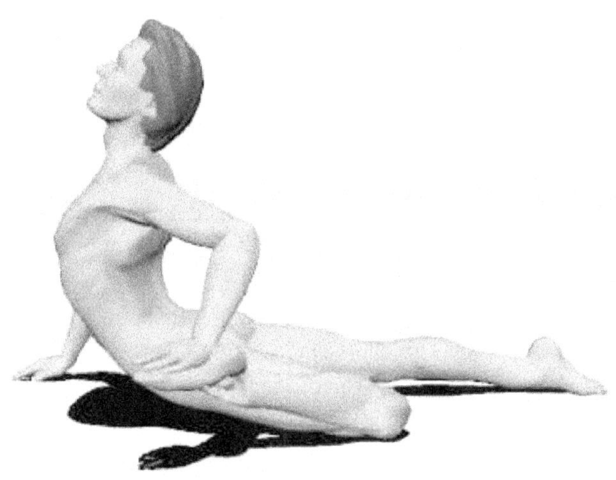

It's difficult to see in the above illustration, but there is a slight twist to the body when you do the half frog pose. The side with the foot will raise slightly, and this will tweak the spine, and it will make a world of difference in your pose.

The organs located around the stomach are going to be quite happy, for they like being stretched.

The back is going to be singing, and the hips and thighs are going to be quite open. Nice.

Take your time doing this, be careful of the knee. No force, just relax your way into it.

GREEN BELT

Two thirds of the way there. It's really happening, isn't it? You are making great progress, and you are becoming aware of yourself as the source of awareness by leaps and bounds.

Of course, being two/thirds of the way up the mountain, the roughest third is right ahead of you.

But, by now you have realized that you have to spend some time doing this, and you have to be regular and dedicated and never miss a yoga session.

The good news...you don't want to miss a session because it is so darned fun.

Isn't it interesting? Did you ever think that just sitting in the same spot, making a few moves, stretching and twisting your body, could be so much fun?

But, underneath the fun of the body is the growing awareness, the developing spirituality.

That is what is truly driving you.

There is just something so darned nice about being you.

Okay, enough chit chat. No more breaks, no more patting yourself on the back...it's time to break out the pitons and spikes and start to really climb up the coming the steep walls.

Rock and roll, baby. We're almost to the home stretch!

YOUR FIFTH MEDITATION

Fix your attention.

Fix your Attention, that is, focus your awareness...the awareness that is you...on an object.

See how long you can prolong your attention.

One object, no thoughts, except perhaps the one question, 'What are you?'

Obviously, you are increasing your power, and you are learning a very precise method that will enable you to move through this world with impunity, and to accomplish anything you want.

You may do this in any posture.

We usually don't fix attention on our bodies or anything in them. Your intent is to get out of the body, not lose yourself in the workings of the body.

In the martial arts, BTW, we practice fixing our attention by putting out candles by punching at them, and stopping an inch or two short. Interesting, eh?

POSTURE SIXTY-ONE
Eka Pada Rajakapotasana II (One-Legged King Pigeon Pose II)

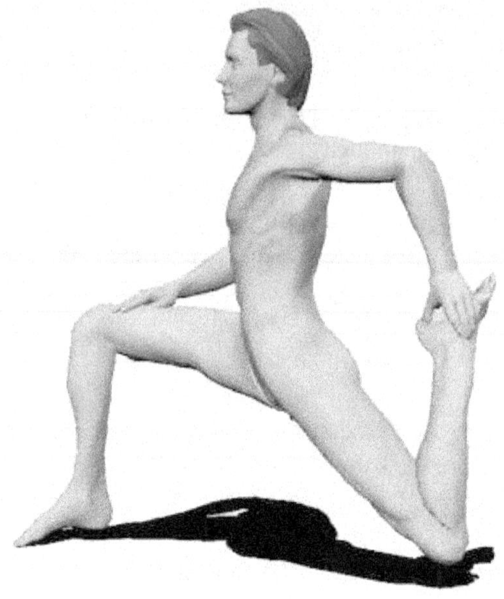

The One Legged King Pigeon Pose 2 will stretch the back and the hip flexors, and will improve posture greatly. On the healthy side, it massage the abdominal organs.

The main thing here is creating balance in an unorthodox position. I was a soft knee when I started this, and did it on a pillow for a few weeks. Then I finally grunted up and overcame.

And, once the balance kicked in, it was very enjoyable. Actually, it was very enjoyable feeling the muscles twitch back and forth while seeking balance, but I was thinking about the knee. Silly me.

THE JUDGING MIND

As one separates from a knowledge of the self as awareness, and from the Greater Awareness, there occurs a deeply felt spiritual pain.

To not know oneself is to deny oneself is to be a thing rather than a spirit.

Now, when one feels this great pain, one starts creating the universe as a place of pain.

This is why there is war and disease and the vast plethora of attitudes and methods that cause all of mankind such incredible misery.

This explains why the person who thinks he is a body is so apt to betray and hurt a person who knows he is a spirit.

The person who knows he is a spirit reminds the unaware being of his separation and of his pain, thus, the unaware strike back at that (the spirit) which causes him so much pain.

It doesn't matter that he is causing it to himself, he is unaware, and just creating his own universe, and, in this case, perpetuating and making ever larger his own misery.

So, choose your friends wisely.

And, don't judge others, lest you be judged yourself, and made to pay in pain and misery.

POSTURE SIXTY-TWO
Salamba Sirsasana (Supported Headstand)

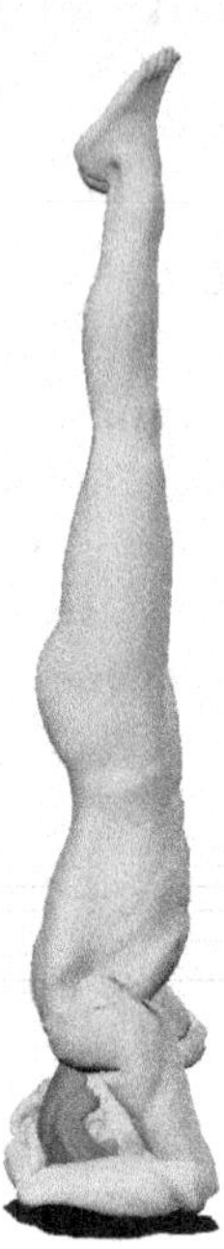

Inversions, love 'em!

You can use a blanket to pad the head, and you can balance up against a wall, when you begin this one. And don't forget to spread the weight out along the forearms so everything is as comfy as possible.

Now, everything being upside down, the body is going to love the reverse settling of the blood.

The brain, in particular is going to feel great, and this includes such glands as the pituitary and pineal.

And, the twitching back and forth of the muscles, upside down, is going to be quite different from the right side up version, and this is going to result in a body vibration, very subtle, that stays with you all day.

POLITICS AND OTHER FALSE GODS

Human beings go into motor, create tension through push/pull, with everything they see.

They can't remember why they exist, you see, and so are constantly seeking for stability. Going into motor with things, even stupid things like bug bites, causes an experience which tends to cement (in the worst sense of the word) the human existence.

Now, one of the things humans do is build machines.

Well, yeah, machines are good, right?

But people build machines of human relationships. Like corporations and governments and institutions. Yikes!

Now, on the face of it, there is nothing wrong with this practice. And if mankind wasn't so severely tainted and corrupted, things like machines (institutions, corporations, governments, etc.) would be fine and dandy.

I'm all for easy living.

But, the unaware human being joins a group of this ilk in exchange for enhancement of power.

Power is a corruption of the whole self.

And, the machine tends to replace the lost image of God, or Greater Awareness.

A cop says, "You can't do that!" And, he is the authority. He has established himself above you, so he is better than you, which, in a terrible and corrupted sense, makes him feel...better.

So we end up worshipping this bizarre configurations of machines, and they are but false gods, replacement for our lost Greater Awareness.

You worship a politician with cheers and votes, and yet he does the same old same old, betraying the public trust, elevating himself.

You worship corporate presidents with admiration and money.

Heck, even religious institutions have gone down this terrible bramble path.

When a church is more interested in the accumulation of money, artifacts, icons, and other things that represent the real world, then they have forsaken the spiritual world, and of what use are they then?

But I will leave you to judge the worth of your religion, or any institution, for yourself...simply make two columns on a sheet of paper. Write down in one column the good things the institution does, and in the other, the bad things. And make sure you list the betrayals and lies, or the completed and beneficial promises, in the columns.

POSTURE SIXTY-THREE
Pasasana (Noose Pose)

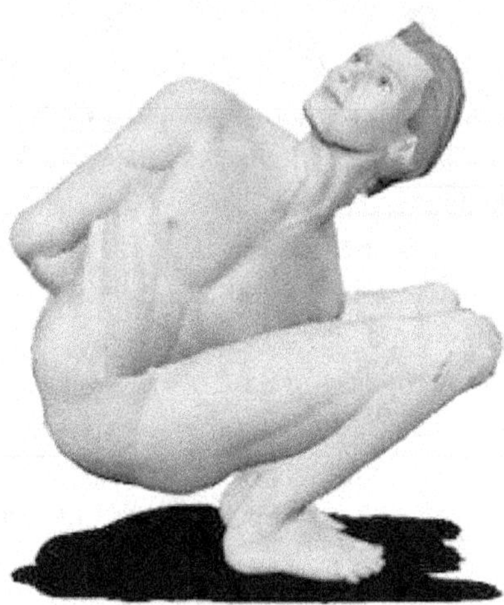

There are many variations on this cool pose. Pictured is a simple one. However, you can go simpler by putting the hands in the prayer pose. You can go more difficult by looping the down arm (the left one in the picture) around the knees and then around to the back.

The hands are clasped in the back. When is really wild is to put them in the prayer position between the shoulder blades while doing this posture.

Be careful if you have back injuries. That aside, you are going to see a plethora of benefits (indeed, the more difficult the poses it often seems the more benefits!) including intestines and bladder and kidneys and spine and so on and so on.

Relax. Breath. Enjoy.

THE POSITIVE ASPECT OF SELF-ASSERTION

It is not enough that one be the center of the universe, one must believe they are the center of the universe!

This gets interesting when one considers that this holds true for every human being on earth.

You see, you must act as if you are the center of the universe, all while allowing every single other human being to be the center of the universe.

Interesting problem, eh?

Yet, as you delve into this, you will find that an inner discipline of life arises. You will find a code of conduct in all your affairs just begging to be implemented.

This is one of those things you keep finding out about and finding out about, and one day...everybody around you is happy.

They respect you and cherish you as the center of the universe, this solely for the reason that you have cherished them as the center of the universe.

Talk about making the universe mirror your inner thoughts!

Being self assertive is not being a hard charger, it is merely being the center of activity. Even as you move through a crowd and remain the center, will all the centers shift to respect you.

POSTURE SIXTY-FOUR
Pasasana (Noose Pose)

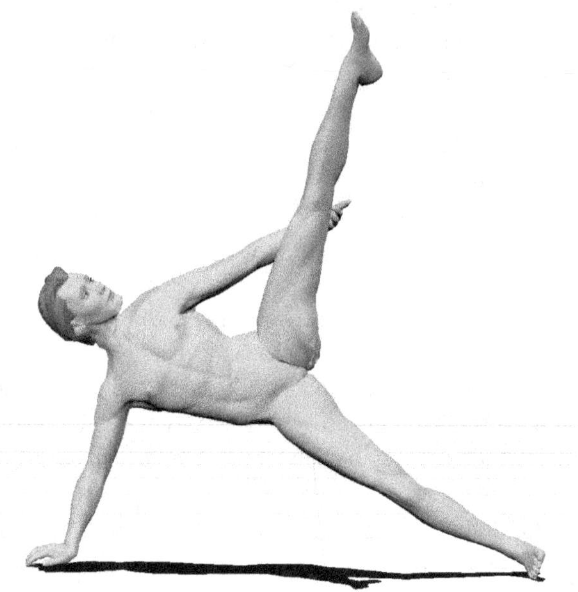

By now you should be pushing on the extremes of the side plank. Here is one version. See how high you can grab the leg, until you can grab the big toe.

This one is going to shiver your timbers, mainly, make you work the side muscles until you create balance.

Relax. Breath. Enjoy.

DEFEATING DICHOTOMY

To understand duality, or dichotomy, or bipoloar disorders, or schizophrenia, or republican and democrat, or good and evil, or any other such term or terms, one need merely understand that there are two terminals to the motor.

Two terminals, and each terminal can push or pull.

A human being can lose sight of his own nature to the extent that he thinks that he is one of the terminals. So, for instance, he becomes a Republican. This obsesses him, but it also makes him function, and gives him reason for existence.

But the truth is that the universe is held together by the tension between the motors, and thus, at heart, the human being knows that he is contributing to the furtherance of the universe by holding to one or the other of the terminals. And he knows that there are times when he must shift to the other terminal to keep the balance.

Everybody knows Russia invented baseball, right?
Yet, baseball was invented in the United States.
This is the balance between east and west.
This is two terminals racing to a tension.

Okay, too far fetched for you. Try this one.

If a good man arises, a bad man will arise to oppose him. This keeps the motor in balance, and keeps the universe afloat.

Weird, eh?

And the solution would be not to stamp out evil, but to understand that if you didn't have somebody shouting out good, you wouldn't have somebody shouting out evil.

And the opposite is also true.

But, to be honest, good or bad, beauty or evil, republican or democrat, it is all a judgement, an opinion, an evaluation, and therefore it has no basis in fact.

So the Democrats rise up and the Republicans wane, and the waveform of the universe, the vibration that has crest and trough in the affairs of man, swings back and forth, and the Republicans rise up and the Democrats wane.

And so on.

As the balance swings one way or the other, people will shift from terminal to terminal to keep the universe (their lives) in a semblance of balance.

The essence of life is to keep motors functioning, to keep terminals in opposition, that man might have existence. And this on the smallest level to the highest magnitude...from atoms to universes...from the fight for survival to kid's games to the highest workings of philosophy or government or economics or whatever.

A crueler trap could not be imagined.
Yet, one can live in motor, and be enlightened, and not be trapped.
Of course, one has to be educated as to their own spiritual nature.

POSTURE SIXTY-FIVE
Utthita Hasta Padangustasana (Extended Hand-To-Big-Toe Pose)

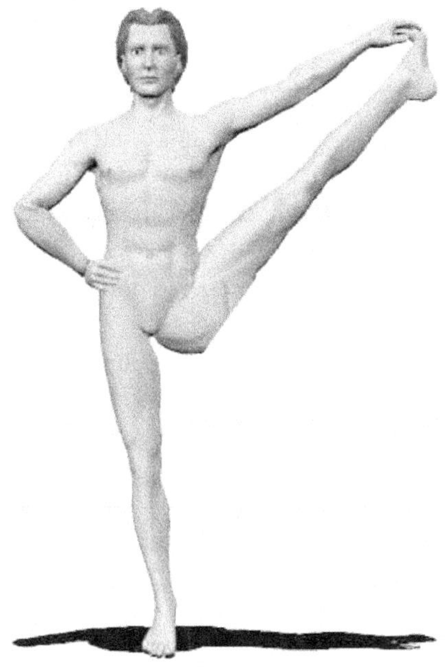

Now we're having fun. Just lift that leg and grab the toe.

You are going to stretch out those hips and have a wonderful sense of balance once you get this standing big toe pose down.

This pose, all postures that utilize the leg in such manner, are going to build leg strength and core strength.

Remember, body energy comes from the tan tien, so breath as if to the center, and let the energy course through your body.

DEFEATING HINDRANCES

Here is the problem: one is naturally drawn towards the universe, for the universe offers existence, and therefore life.

Well, heck, you like living, don't you?

But, to hold to yourself (or go to yourself) as a spiritual being, you must defeat that natural draw when it is tainted by hindrances.

So, when you feel the desire to own many things, and you know it is an attachment (a motor) that is not doing you any good, simply go in the other direction: give things away.

And, when you feel the urge to drink, go in the opposite direction. Take a long, sober walk.

Look, it is merely setting up a counterbalance to your tilting universe that you might stay balanced.

And, heck, be creative in setting up your counterbalances. I mean, no reason why you can't have fun with this, right?

Want to drink? Good. Make yourself a drink, then drive a hundred miles out into the desert, climb a mountain, and drink.

Don't get in a big fight with yourself, merely find a way to let the positives and the negatives fight, and go out and enjoy yourself.

But, if you are unable to make your counterbalance work, you should sit in posture and consider the good and the bad of whatever demon you are falling to.

What are the good things drink does...what are the bad?

You see, things, life, is not good or bad, and sometimes you try too hard, and this sets up your own resistance to your cure.

So don't take the good and bad viewpoint, merely view whatever is happening as it is.

POSTURE SIXTY-SIX
Upavistha Konasana (Wide-Angle Seated Forward Bend)

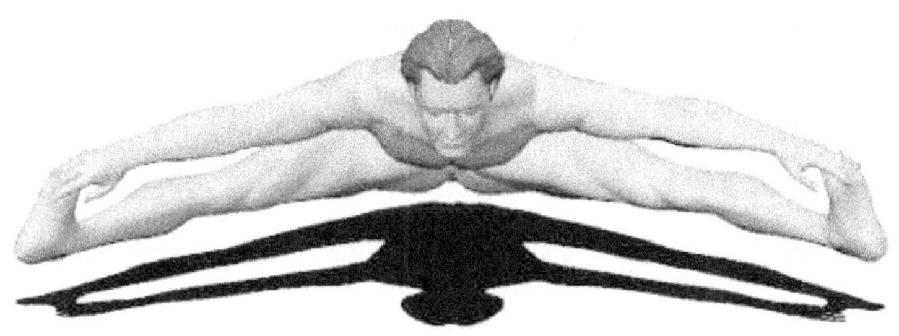

Now this is one of those stances you should have been working on long, and perhaps I should have put it earlier in the book. But, here it is. Half way between the splits, and a forward bend. The best of both worlds.

The hips will open, the waist will bend, and you can just enjoy the peace and quiet of your own mind.

PLAYING THE UNIVERSE

The universe is comprised of atoms, which atoms have three essential parts, the proton, the electron, and the neutron.

The proton is positive, and the electron is negative, and the neutron is merely there. Doesn't do anything. Does...nothing.

That's the way life is.

You have people who play aggressive, are always on the charge (attack), are described as alpha, and so on.

Then you have people who are always in reverse, fearful, do what they are told, are beta, and so on.

That is the majority of people, the billions and billions.

Then you have a handful, probably less than a thousand on the whole planet, who watch, do nothing, sit around, and life works for them.

Now, here is the trick: If a person sits around and life doesn't work for them, then they aren't neutronic, they are so electronic that they aren't functioning. They need a protonic person to come along and kick their butt into gear. They will actually sit on the couch and watch TV until the world comes crashing down upon them, and then they will wander the streets, stealing, and telling all who will listen that life is terrible and the it's all the politicians' faults and...do you get the idea?

But if a person sits around and life works, that is neutronic. And here we are talking about a person who either has innate and powerful abilities, or we are talking about a person who knows that he is (has studied scripture and done yoga), and who can do (has done martial arts until he understands and can handle and manipulate the force and the flows of the universe with ease), and is not sucked into the protonic/electronic flow of the universe (asceticism).

Now, the funny thing about this whole thing is this...the functioning Neutronic Being has presence. He walks into a room where the Protonic person is being overly aggressive with an electronic person, that action will suddenly stop.

If he walks into a room where somebody is sobbing and crying, going too electronic, that person will immediately adhere to the Neutronic person, and within a few words, maybe even just the brush of Neutronic presence, the electronic person will stop whining and moaning.

The neutronic person provides a balance for the protonic and electronic motion of the universe.

And here is the only way to understand this.

The universe is a play for the neutronic person.

The proton chases and the electron runs away solely for the benefit of the Neutron.

In other words, the universe is here to entertain me.

If I get sucked into action, I betray my own spiritual neutronicity, and to that degree I am ineffective, and protonic or electronic myself.

To the degree that I hold to my Neutronicity, in spite of all accusations of Fabianism, to that degree will I have magnitude and effect the play of the universe and bring balance to the universe.

And, by I, I mean you.

Interesting, eh?

POSTURE SIXTY-SEVEN
Pincha Mayurasana (Feathered Peacock Pose)

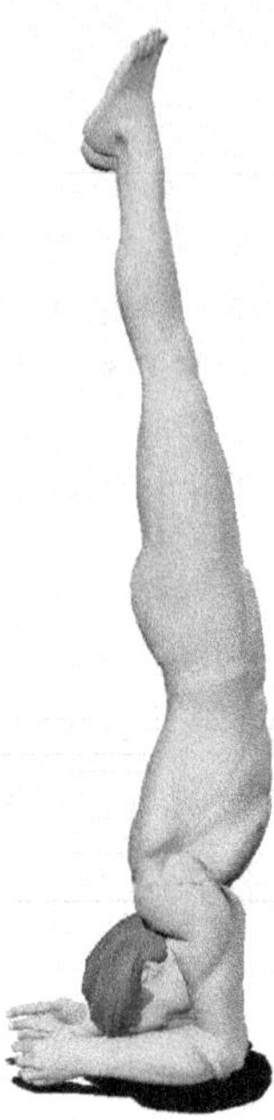

This pose is like the supported headstand (Salamba Sirsasana), but a couple of inches higher, with the arms a little more forward.

You'll get much the same benefits as in the supported headstand, but you'll also get more balance, finer balance, and more control

Onward, and ever upward.

THE FOURFOLD PATH

Now, there is one point I should bring up, and it is why there is a certain disjointedness to this tome, a certain awkwardness, and even why there are certain small discrepancies.

Heck, there is even, on the surface, contradictions. Until one realizes that sometimes I am making a point from one terminal, or another, or from above, or from within the machine itself.

That is to say that the point of view of each of the four disciplines, monk, yogi, martial artist, ascetic, coming from a different position in relation to the motor, the terminals therein, or the action of, sometimes seem to contradict, until you take into account that they are coming from different positions in the motor.

I am writing from the viewpoint of four different disciplines, and these disciplines take place at different points in life.

Speaking from the human body point of view.

The young Turk learns martial arts, the baby learns yoga (ever see a baby suck its toe? Tell me that isn't perfect Yoga!) The old monk studies scripture when he can no longer move around (old people reading the bible in a last ditch effort to understand what comes next!) The ascetic, bruised from war, negates the world that led him to that ultimate frustration.

And, age doesn't necessarily define these disciplines (a monk could be young, a yogi can be old, and so on), but there is still a timeline in which somebody would study these things.

The ideal timeline would be do Yoga while studying scripture, learn martial arts while studying scripture so that one may manipulate the world, refuse to have dealings with the world when one needs a bit extra study of scripture.

Do you understand the problem in this tome?

The problem is not just that I am blending four discipline which come from different viewpoints (be it of the same motor), the problem is that I am taking the whole timeline, the viewpoint of the beginner to the intermediate to the advanced to the expert to the master, and presenting it all in one volume!

Thus, I shift between yogic viewpoint to neutronic viewpoint to scriptural viewpoint to frugal viewpoint to...and all the viewpoints come from different times of a lifetime.

Sheesh. What a mess!

But, truth, I ain't doin' such a bad job.

The point here is to give you a solid feel for how everything comes together, how each discipline can support the other, and how we aren't arriving at different goals, but rather same one, all while twining out paths.

To be honest, while I am doing a good job, one should study all of my work, the martial arts and the yoga and neutronic scripture...and then apply it to the classical scripture and the classical modes of discipline.

Look, when I present Matrixing to Martial Artists I tell them that matrixing is a logic, and they must apply it to their life.

And this path I take, this Fourfold Path, I describe it to you, but your experience is going to be unique. And you have to figure out where on the path you are, whether you need more study in yoga or martial arts or economical life living or whatever, or less, or whatever.

I am describing a path, a path that has been split in four over the ages, and kept that way by fanatics and true believers.

I am telling you that you must be true believer in assembling the original knowledge back into the whole picture.

I describe, but you live, and this tome is nothing more than direction for you to choose from according to your need.

POSTURE SIXTY-EIGHT
Ustrasana (Camel Pose)

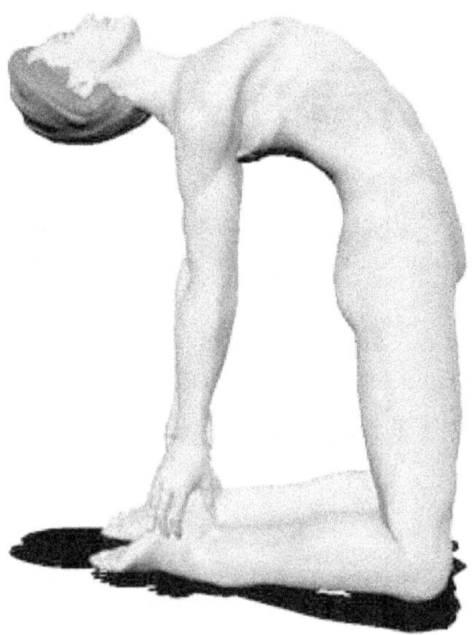

The Camel Pose is a wonderful back bend, it stretches the chest and causes all sorts of good things to happen in lung and kidney and digestion and so on.

This pose is similar to the Bow Pose, but requires a bit of balance.

As you get better with this pose, close your eyes and let your attention, and imagination, wander upwards.

It is a big sky above you, and it is all yours!

FEEDING THE MOTOR

Now here is the thing, when you join a machine, you are contributing life force to a group of people, to a concept, to a motor of life force that permeates the universe.

You go to work for a company, and you get a bit of prestige and recognition for your contribution to that company.

You join a bigger company, you get more perks, more life force back for the investment of life force put in. Last out that company long enough, make large enough contribution to that company, and you could be Pope, or President, or Chairman of the Board, or whatever.

If you are an entertainer the machine isn't always so tight, more potential for flame out, but if you succeed, the life force back, the fame and the glamour, it is something sizable.

I joined two motors.

I joined writers, which is art, which gives much reward, but the risk, and so on.

And, I joined martial artists, and here is where things get interesting.

A martial Artist doesn't just give to his group machine, he gives to the group of his machine throughout time.

Most companies have a curve, they rise, they flourish, they wane, they fall, no more company. So the life force you put into that company...disappears. Machine gone. So you move on to another company, another escapade, and it waxes and wanes, and is gone.

And you are vagabond through the ages, joining and finding yourself out of life force work and...and that's the way it goes.

So you join something more lasting, like a political party. Political parties last longer than companies. Sort of. Except when you consider that political parties are machines, and their curve is longer, but the curve is liable to twist in some weird belief system (communism, Marxism, whatever) at any moment. Or just be revolted into oblivion.

Okay, had enough, so you join a church. But, even if they last a few millennium, churches rise and fall, there is the constant influx of belief systems to keep everything unsettled, and so on.

And all this is the history of planet earth. A series of machines/corporations/political parties/movements/etcetera that wax and wane.

So I got tired of the machine method for having existence, and I started my own church, and that church is based on me. And you can only join it is you believe...not in me...but in you.

I am the center of the universe. I am God. And to the degree that you believe that you are the center of the universe, that you are God, to that degree you can be in my religion.

And the catechism of this religion is Neutronics, which is based on an understanding of the motor of the universe, and of the reality of you.

And it is proof against any temporary fad or belief system, because the one question you must ask is...does that fad or belief system support me as the center of the universe.

Only if you start believing that somebody else doesn't have the right and duty to consider themselves as the center of the universe, will this church fail.

If somebody hurts somebody else, is that believing that somebody else has the right to be the center of the universe?

Look, the point is this: when it comes to writing, I don't want to write for a temporary place on a best seller list. I want people to pick up my books in a thousand years and get excited, find relevance, find themselves.

And, when it comes to martial arts: there is a life force permeating this universe, and this life force has been contributed to by every single person who has bowed himself onto a mat, and it is tapped upon by every single person who has ever thrown a punch.

It is the chi of the martial arts, and it is an actual life force, kept in place by the beings who contribute to it, and it exists through the ages, and it is to this that I belong.

Not to a machine or a corporation, for they deal in temporary things, rewards so you can buy houses and cars.

The martial art has a spirit, and anybody can tap into it, but not for houses and cars and piles of cash, rather for health and calmness and peace of mind and the ability to look any man in the eye and believe in him.

Do you understand what I belong to?
And, it is perfectly fine with me if you don't.

POSTURE SIXTY-NINE
Natarajasana (Lord of the Dance Pose)

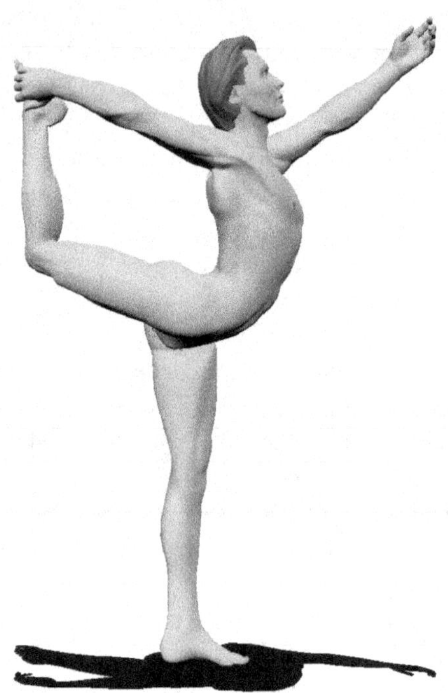

The Lord of the Dance Pose. The ultimate in balance and stretch and flexibility.

Note how the top shin goes up. See how the arms are split in Y.

This is looking forever and meaning it!

This is going to work the whole body, and the whole body is going to benefit from it.

And this means that you are going to tap into cosmic energy with a vengeance!

Welcome.

YOUR DUTY

As you progress, as you elevate yourself to your natural state of spirituality, you must be careful of those around you.

And, as you grow larger, you must be careful in an ever widening circle.

Look, as you rid yourself of hindrances, take control of your motors, something interesting happens.

When you have no motors tugging you out of balance, when your mind is calm and empty, when you see unhindered the reality of All, nature abhors a vacuum.

You don't generate static, so the denizens of the universe will want to inject their static into you.

Choose your friends wisely.

Either they will fall into you, moaning and whining of their plight, or they will speak ill of you, not understanding that they are just speaking ill of themselves, they are just projecting, and looking for a place to project, their unhappiness.

And, simply avoid the ignorant, except as you may instruct them.

You have the glow of wisdom. Somewhere in their boxed up, little nature, they see that truth, and they know it is theirs, and they want it, but they don't know how to loosen their bonds, they don't know how to get what you have.

So, avoid as you must, and protect yourself, and instruct as you can, depending on circumstance that you remain protected and above the fray.

Really, walking the Fourfold Path I prescribe is like walking on a single 2 by 4 through a stadium filled with animals that like your scent and wish to fight over you.

Still, as you grow in Awareness, as you become aware of the Awareness of All, as you encourage the growth of Awareness in all, you have a duty, a responsibility, to share that Awareness.

If you don't, the 2 by 4 will fall, and you will be devoured by those who love you.

POSTURE SEVENTY
Parsvottanasana (Intense Side Stretch Pose)

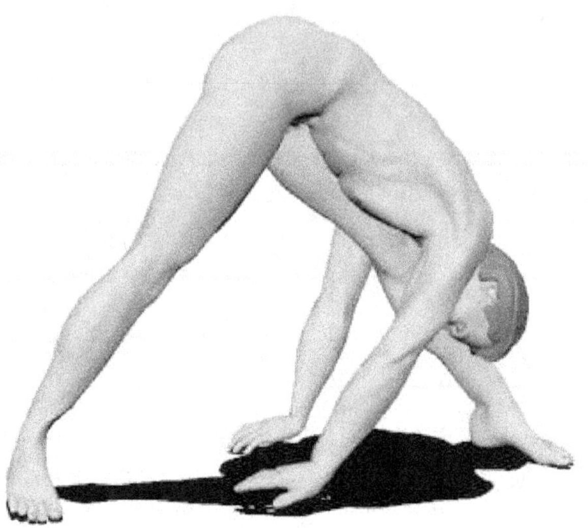

The intense side stretch is going to pull them hamstrings tighter than a cat gut fiddle.

So, relax. You know the benefits. You know the supreme feeling of glow and satisfaction and long life when you do this pose, so just relax them hams, and let it happen!

The only thing that stands in the way of you is...you.

So get out of the way!

Remember, get in a fight with yourself...and somebody is going to lose!

CREATION

Your life is an act of creation; you create your life every moment of every day.

When you learn a discipline, such as Yoga, martial arts, or whatever, that discipline should be founded on scientific principle.

However, there must be room within that science for art.

There is an art to applying science.

There is a science to applying art.

Thus, when I instruct people I encourage them to hold true to the scientific principles, but I tell them they must use those principles to create.

In this book I am giving you 90 postures, with a few extra here and there, and a bit of advice about creating advanced variations, and so on.

However, if you read the rather wondrous tome 'Asanas: 608 Yoga Poses,' by Dharma Mittra, there are 608 poses.

The point is that Yoga is learned, through discipline, but at some point the student must demonstrate his own creativity. He must become the inventor of Yoga.

Thus, one creates poses.

Some of the poses are better meditation; some of the poses are for body; some of the poses are for the Greater Awareness.

It doesn't matter what the poses are or do, what matters is that you get the discipline well enough that you can extend it, make it larger.

And, as time flows, poses will be lost. And discovered again. And lost.

So the message is this. As you seek a Greater Awareness, don't forget to seek through creative posing.

POSTURE SEVENTY-ONE
Tiptoe Pose (Prapadasana)
Squat Prayer

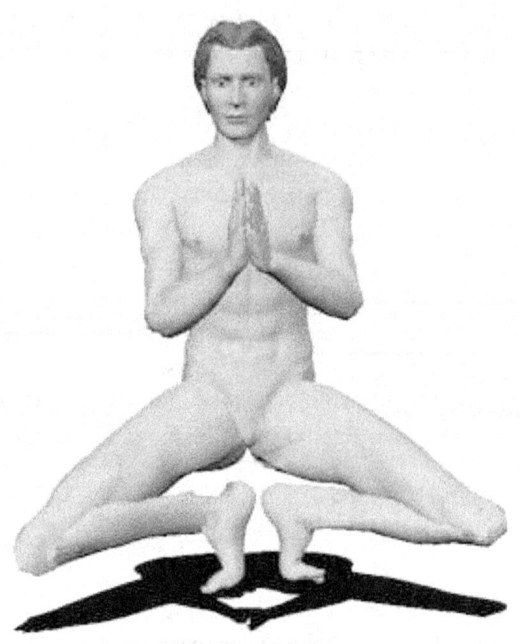

Squat Prayer, as I call it, is a difficult one for my software. One should actually be sitting on the heels, with the heels touching one another.

That said, the balancing act in your ankles and feet is going to bring them to full power.

This is a nice one for calm meditation.

Relax. Breath. Enjoy.

REMAINING TRUE TO THE PATH

To the degree that you hold to your determination, to the degree that you persist, to the degree that you do not allow yourself to be swayed...to that degree will you succeed.

To succeed means to life as it is, in true lights, to be immune to shadow play, be it generated by yourself or others.

Still, the greatest growth comes when you teach others.

When you take something you have earned through hard work and dedication and give it to somebody, you get a greater something in return.

Often, you don't know what it is, will be, but the truth is this, when it comes to the Fourfold Path, the more you give away the more you accumulate.

When it comes to your being the truth is this: the more you shine the light of truth that is you, the brighter you become.

Or, to borrow from The Tao (one of my favorite quotes, and made into one of the 24 Neutronic Principles: 'Do nothing until nothing is left undone.'

Look, the truth is this:

A yogi will increase awareness into his own body, and use that to springboard himself into the greater body of awareness.

A martial artist will increase awareness of force and flow, and that being all the universe is made of, will become a master of the universe.

A monk will study the scripture of Greater Awareness, until he is that greater awareness.

An ascetic will denounce the universe, until all that is left is awareness.

And, one who studies all four methods will benefit fourfold, and come to understand the whole path four times faster.

It is true.

POSTURE SEVENTY-TWO
Three Point Landing

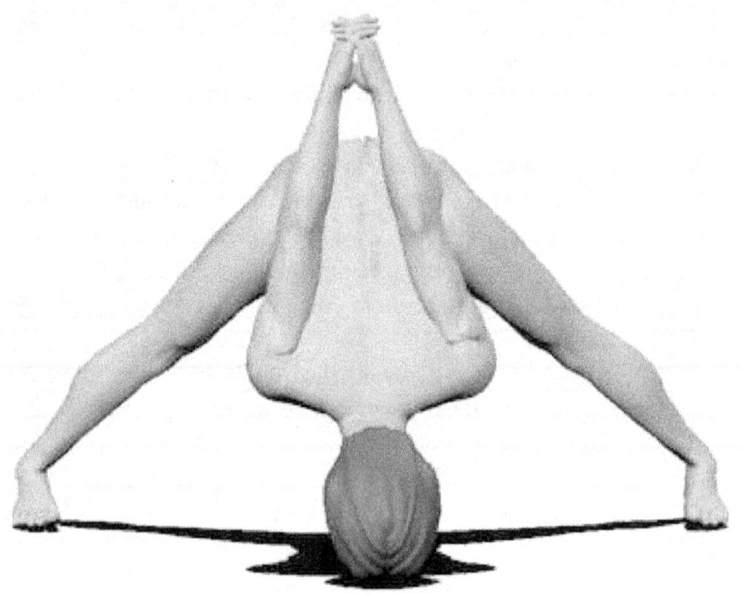

I call this Three Point Landing, and once you have landed, it is very restful.

Actually it is a variation of the Wide Legged Forward Bend, Prasarita Padottanasana. Or, perhaps this is the pose and Prasarita Padottanasana is the variation. No matter. What's in a name, eh?

Anyway, the difference here is that this one doesn't use hands. Your neck will become strong and enduring.

Rest. Breath. Enjoy.

WHAT'S IN A NAME?

I mean, really!

A rose by any other name...nothing could be as lovely as a tree...and so on.

The point is this, when you create something that has never been, there is no name for it, and thus, there is Russian Graffiti all over the backside of the moon, but a crater is still a lovely crater no matter what you call it.

When you name something, you are giving it reference.

But a snap kick in Karate is the same as a snap kick in Kung Fu is the same as a snap kick in...any other art.

So the name is important as a reference point, but it is unimportant in relation to understanding the concept behind the name.

When you speak of OM, or kiai, or some other utterance of the spirit, you are talking about transmittal of awareness without the sound.

So how do you describe a sound that isn't? Except to say...the will to project an idea without vocalization.

And, how do you describe yourself, the real awareness, except to say it can't be seen, felt or encountered by any perception.

And, God is a concept that cannot be described in words.

Because you can't describe the fact of awareness, except to say that between the universes that are spiritual beings there are encounters, and these encounters make up the physical world.

POSTURE SEVENTY-THREE
Elbow Lunge

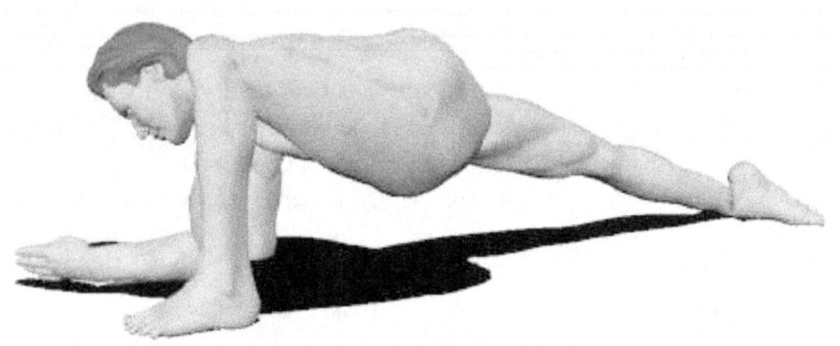

I call this one the elbow lunge. Got to be a regular name for it. You should probably look for it. Good excuse to do a little yoga browsing. You learn so much by learning what other people are doing. The trick is to separate the dope from the genius. Interesting task. And fun, too.

THE SIX FACETS

Okay, this is interesting.

There are Commandments, which would be unbreakable rules (see 'The 24 Principles of Neutronics').

There are Rules, which encourage your behavior amongst your peers. And there are facets, which name I chose so as not to use 'rules' or 'commandments,' and which are sides of the holistic whole that you should be adhering to.

Here they are.

Correct Pose, which is your attitude towards life, which should be to be balanced (Neutronic) as you go forward through time.

Correct Control of the Life Force. Control is everything. Control the body so you can control the mind and be in control of the spirit, and understand the Greater Awareness that substantiates this universe.

Withdrawal, which is to give a certain degree of acceptance to the Ascetic needs of the spirit; to withdraw from your acceptance of the universe to the degree that you realize and grow in Awareness. Be frugal. Be economical. But don't forget to be generous. A miser is never an ascetic.

Attention. Focus Awareness. On an object, on the universe, focus your attention until you see the truth of whatever you are focusing on.

Meditation. Time for yourself. Enhancement of Awareness. You are a universe unto yourself.

Contemplation. Acceptance of what is. Get rid of your rigid attitude; do not judge; accept the universe. If you accept the universe, and don't fight it, your race to enlightenment will happen all that faster.

POSTURE SEVENTY-FOUR
Camatkarasana (Wild Thing)

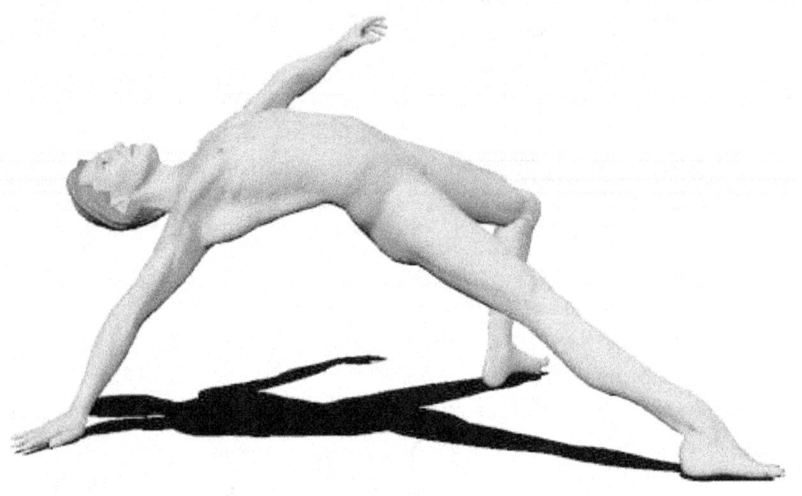

Wild thing. A delicate balancing act. It stretches the back and gives great freedom. What are you looking at up there? Eh? Whatever it is, it's big. That's for sure. Must be you.

THE FIVE PILLARS

You're almost to Brown Belt. Almost to the home stretch. Here are five crucial points you should be implementing into your life.

Don't injure, neither others nor yourself. Don't cause pain or hurt. Do the opposite. Help people. To help people is to help yourself. It is the one selfish act that you are allowed and encouraged to commit.

Be truthful. Don't lie, for that causes a barrier between people. That causes a barrier to Awareness. Not just the Awareness of the other individual, but to the Greater Awareness of All.

Don't steal, not anything, nor any not thing (ideas). There is actually only one crime in this universe, and it is stealing. Every crime can be reduced to the simple act of theft. To commit murder is to steal a life. To commit adultery is to steal a wife. And so on. Just don't steal. And don't let the government steal, either.

Don't be impure. Eat well, sleep well, don't imbibe or take drugs. How can a tainted body accept the discipline of the Fourfold Path? How can a stained mind see the truth of the universe? Of any universe? If you do this, and convince somebody else to do this, and they pay it forward, there will come a time when there is no crime.

Don't covet. If you want something, earn it. Don't dream about it, go get it, but with hard work and your stalwart character intact.

POSTURE SEVENTY-FIVE
Adho Mukha Vrksasana (Handstand)

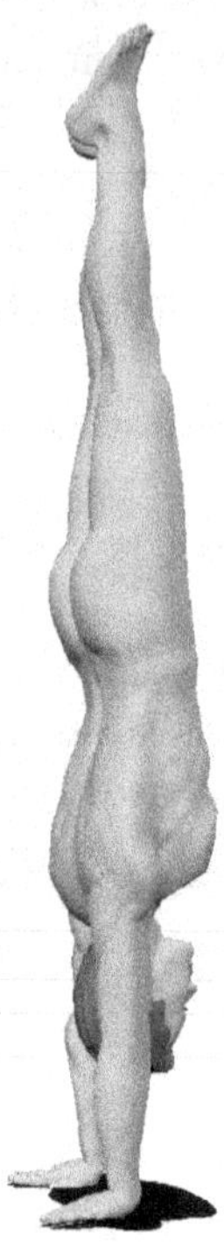

The handstand. Great for the arms, and balance, and opening the door to all sorts of things. Like doing the splits while in a hand stand. Like doing push ups in a hand stand. Like...there is no end to the amount of fun you can have doing a simple handstand!

BROWN BELT

Oh! Good Lard! You've made it to Brown Belt! You are the most magnificent lion to EVER roar in the jungle! And I mean it!

Now, a caution: there are two places where people drop out. At the beginning, or else right at the stretch before the finishing line.

So, rededicate yourself. Set your sights on accomplishing those last few asanas.

Listen, you are climbing the steepest part, the face of the cliff right before the pinnacle. All you have to do is dig in those toes, claw those fingers, and pull yourself up!

Look! It's right there! Above you! A few grabs and you've made it!

Do you feel that coming sense of satisfaction?

Do you feel the sense of accomplishment about to overwhelm you?

How could you dream of anything except making those last few feet to the summit?

How?

I tell you this...what you are about to do has been done by few.

A few people in Yoga, a few people in martial arts, a few monks and ascetics...that's all!

You see, the Fourfold Path has never been seen before. I matrixed it out of the parts. And while many people have walked a single path to the top, very few have walked a single path and seen the whole presented by four paths brought together!

Go on, look at yourself. Brighter, with more smarts than you ever knew you had!

Go on. Make it. The universe will be brighter for the life force you are about to contribute!

YOUR SIXTH MEDITATION

Imagine you are in space.
There are no objects, not even a floor to sit upon.
There is no gravity.

I took away my body
and floated out in a space
absent of all friends
where went the human race

I took away the planet
on which I stood and spun
I watched the stars unwind
the heavens came undone

I took away the Gods
thoughts of heav'n and hell
and time became a murmur
and I became a swell

I became a particle
a wave that gave no light
I knew at last I'd found
the dark eternal night

POSTURE SEVENTY-SIX
Padangusthasana (Big Toe Pose)

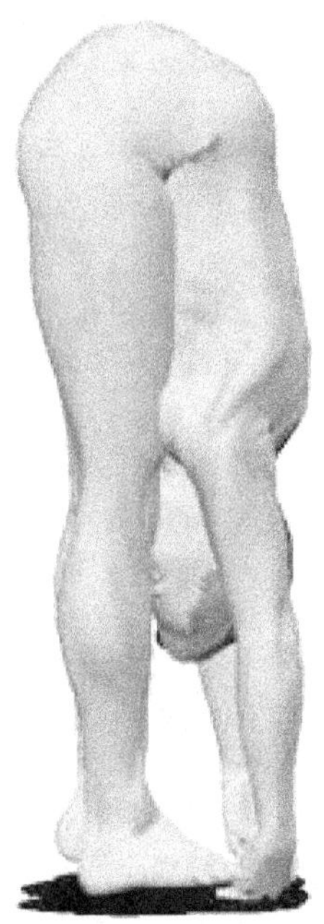
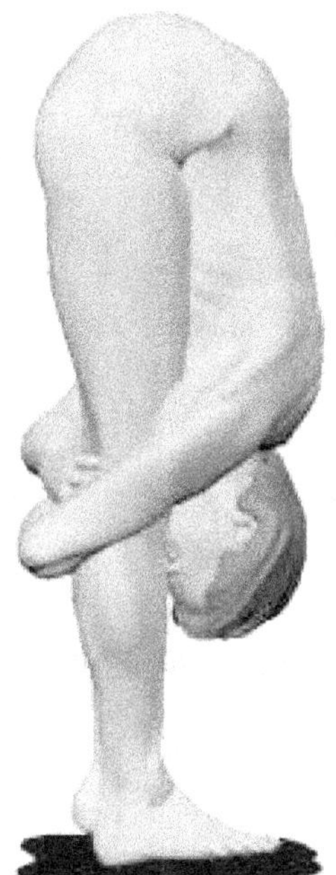

The Big Toe Pose, in which one folds at the waist (notice the lack of bend in the back) and holds the big toe.

Actually, I prefer hugging the knees, as in the pic on the right. The reason is that I prefer to hold onto myself as an anchor, it gives me stability, and allows me to relax in body while the arms do their duty.

Obviously, you are going to get flexibility out of this asana, and you are going to improve the kidneys, digestion, the lungs, the whole nine yards.

Don't forget to bend the other way, to find an asana that bends the back the other way.

MATRIXING 101

Slowly but surely you move through poses. And, by Matrixing, you make sure that examine the viability of linking one pose to all other poses.

It's easy if, in the beginning, you just choose four or so poses and put them on a graph and do all the combos, X-ing off the ones that don't work well, and making a list of those that do work well.

Of course, you may remember that book I mentioned that has 608 yoga poses in it.

Imagine a matrix 608 poses across the top, and 608 poses down the side. Good Lard! You'd have (count fingers and toes) 369,664 changes of posture!

And that's not counting things like which side goes to which side, deviations and variations, and so on!

Do you understand why the study of Yoga is a study in the infinite? Of infinity?

Let's see, if you were adept at all poses, and began doing every link, and it took you one minute to accomplish, that's 369,664 minutes to do all yoga!

Divided by 60 minutes, it would take you a little over 6,000 hours to do all of Yoga!

Or, you could take the 90 poses in this book, do them within a year, have a vast grasp on what Yoga is, and do them all in 135 hours. That's just a five day week with .625 days overtime.

Hey! That's not bad! I guess there's a little Yoga hope out there, after all.

POSTURE SEVENTY-SEVEN
Hanumanasana (Monkey Pose)

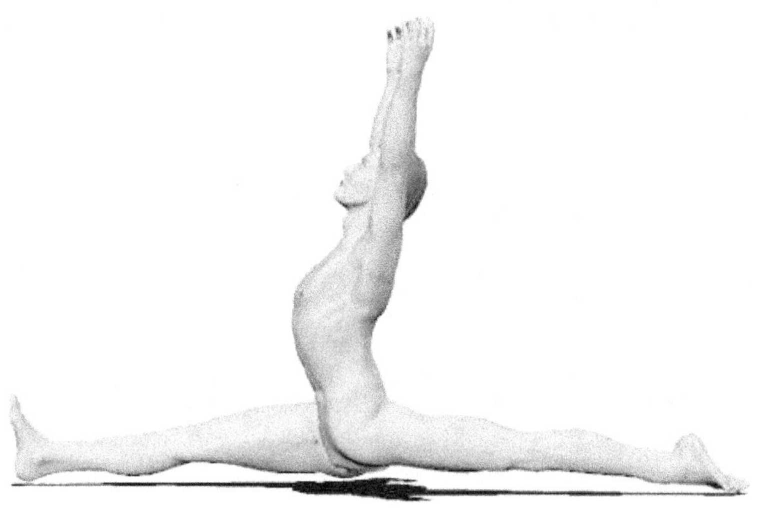

Time for some full splits. You've had a whole book to work towards them, both side and front, so you should be close by now, right?

What? You didn't read this book? You just opened to this page?

Nonsense. Nobody does that. But, if you did, wow!

So, anyway, you should be capable of doing both side splits and front and back splits (as pictured above). The thing to remember, when you do splits, is that you need to take your time, learn how to give messages to the muscles to relax and let go, and learn that you are in charge of the muscles, and that they have to do what you say.

If you can be in charge of the universe of the body, then you can be in charge of the greater universes, such as the mind, or the universe of All.

THE FIVE BODIES

Speaking of the five bodies, or universes, or sheaths, or motors, or whatever you call them, here they are.

The body. A fleshy envelope which all too many people think is the end all be all of life. It is just a body, muscle and bone, and you put them on and take them off like clothes. Uh, that is if you entered your clothes by spiraling down through the neck. That's right, you enter and leave your body by spiraling down through the crown.

If you can't control your body you can't control your emotions.

Emotion. Nobody knows what this one is, and that's why all too many fall to it. Emotion is motion inside the head. In a way, emotions are not real, except to the one generating them. That said, emotions are usually an overflow of vibrations once the life unit becomes overwhelmed. There are emotions that are bad, the cause de-evolution (fear, anger, etc.) And there are emotions that are good: love, joy, etc.

If you can't control your emotions then you can't control your mind.

Mind. A bunch of memory. Control the mind and you have a useful tool. To control the mind one need merely examine reality until he sees that reality is real; that he can discern between reality and that which he thinks is reality in his mind.

If you can't control the mind you can't discover the self (Awareness).

Self. This is the fellow, the 'I am,' the Awareness, that is in charge of mind, emotion and body. The problem is that this fellow generates psychic activities, often calls these activities the mind, and thus, is out of control. Heck, if he is overwhelmed and can't figure out how to fight back, he can create a whole fantasy universe to protect himself. Unfortunately, these fantasy universes don't really protect him, and they become memories that the mind will eventually throw back up at him.

Sort of funny. The mind doesn't really like all this weird gobbledy gook the psychic Awareness throws into it, and it will regurgitate it, often at the worst possible time.

This is why martial arts and matrixing is so useful. Yes, being close to the end of the Yoga you should be thinking in terms of martial arts.

The point is that martial arts make you look at the things of the universe, and analyze them for force and flow, and this makes the person go into reality, and out of the unreality posed by mind and psychic miscalculations and mental malfunction.

If you can't control the self (awareness), then you can't find the Whole Self...the Greater Awareness that is All.

So, five steps. Five steps that make up the whole fourfold path.

Of course, there is more, as the minutiae is immense, and, unfortunately, though understanding the principles is the whole of it, one often can't understand the whole of it until he has dealt with enough minutiae to see the whole picture.

I have, incidentally, detailed how the mind works, how the human being learns, and this is in the book 'Prologue,' which is available at ChurchofMartialArts.com.

POSTURE SEVENTY-EIGHT
Dwi Pada Viparita Dandasana (Upward Facing Two-Foot Staff Pose)

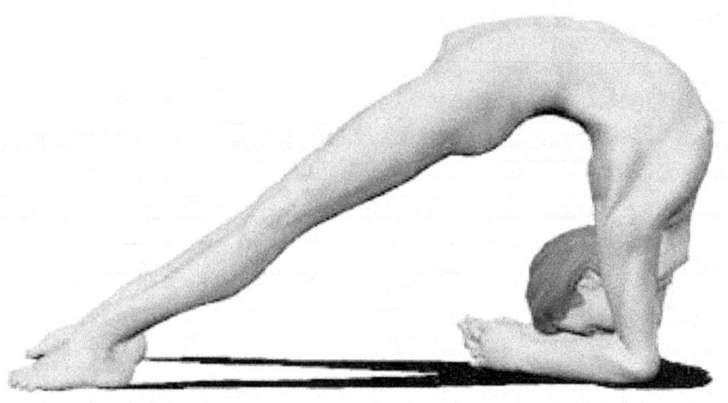

Man, now we are cooking! This is one heck of a great back bend, and it will flex you and stretch you and clean out your innards like nothing else!

Do you notice that I don't bother telling you about benefits and cautions any more? That's because you learned the basics earlier, and you should be applying them.

To not apply what you learn, that's a crime, you know?

YOUR CHOICE

So, you have a choice.

You can believe that you are muscle and bone, hair and sinew, lustful urges and intemperate behavior. Good clean fun, uh?

Or...you can believe that you are not a meat brain looking through eyeballs and listening through ears, the victim of the universe, but, rather a being looking through the eyeballs and ears and such. That you are separate and unique, looking at the show through your perceptions. That if you die you live forever, but that that life is what you create, and it can be heaven, or it can be hell.

Interesting choice, eh?

So, go ahead. Choose.

POSTURE SEVENTY-NINE
Marichyasana I

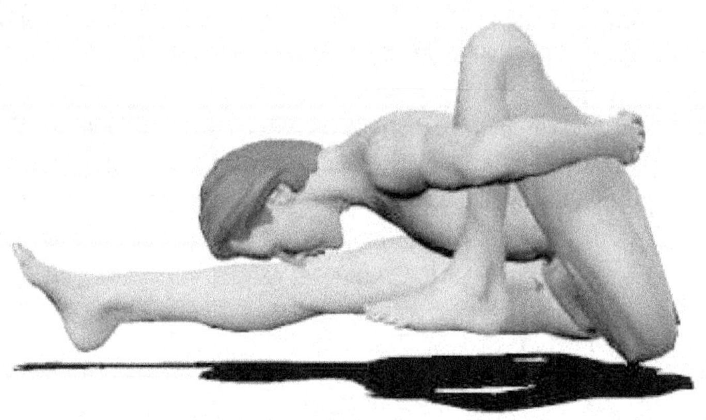

Marichi is considered the father of humanity, and this pose is one heck of a father of all poses. The stretch of the hams, the flex of the head to knee, the binding of the arms. It's all sort of backwards, but creates a forward evolution, if you get what I mean.

Relax. Breath. Enjoy.

THE VIEWPOINT OF A LIBERATED HUNK OF AWARENESS

Now, here is some fun stuff.

Once you view the universe as a liberated hunk of awareness, the universe is different.

Number one, you glow. You glow inside, and you glow outside.

Unfortunately, you are surrounded by a lot of people who don't glow, or who have out of control glow. This means they can't make the universe work. They always have problems and emergencies, and they get themselves in strange fixes, and they always worry about the bills and...and...and so on forever unto the Great Distraction (What I call death.)

For an aware being, however, the universe works. Sometimes he doesn't even seem to do things, but money falls in his lap, the stop lights are always green, ladies appreciate him (but are embarrassed by his presence), and so on.

Number two, the universe glows for an aware being. It is lighter, not so filled with disasters like hurricanes and earthquakes and all that sort of silliness. The universe actually likes the aware being. It likes to be projected (created) by somebody who gives a crap, but gives that crap like it was a big, frothy joke,

Number three, an aware being has S-O-O-O-O-O many more abilities than a meatman.

He can sense what others are thinking. He empathizes with the distraught soul, and his mere presence brings the distraught soul up. He senses when things are going to happen. And here's something really nifty...people who are in the presence of an aware being tend to become more aware themselves, to be happier, and to even share in his heightened abilities.

POSTURE EIGHTY
Krounchasana (Heron Pose)

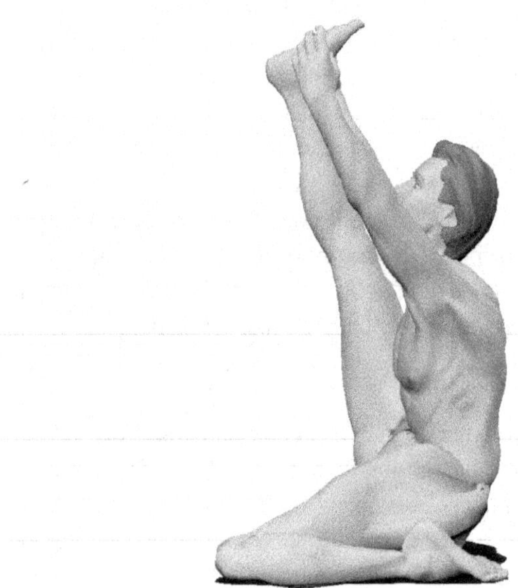

The Heron Pose. A great stretch, a wonderful viewpoint. By now you should feel as innocent as a baby, and you won't worry about what life is going to bring you. You'r in charge. You can control your body, your emotions (except for the joyous ones) are on the wane, your mind is small and reality is pure and shining. Welcome to the real you.

FOR SOMETHING TO BE TRUE....

Okay, so you are a hunk of meat, or at least you think you are, and the universe doesn't work and you're poor and you can't get the things you want...yada yada yada...

Want to know how to make the universe work?

This is a quirky, insidious, little joy I am about to tell you.

So you know how I told you that...

For something to be true the opposite must also be true.

And, you know that the universe is nothing but a big motor.

So, to change the universe, you merely have to change one of the terminals, or one of the push/pull tensions, or, and here it comes, the way you treat, think of, conduct yourself as regards that terminal that motor.

Let's say you're a thief. You steal things. And you have to keep stealing because you never have enough.

But you are stealing things, and you are an Awareness, which can't be measured, and is...a nothing. A Neutron.

So how can a nothing possess a something?

And something will run from nothing because the universe works backwards! It is a projection, and the reverse of what you think it is, which is the controlling factor in your life!

But if you push things away, then they will start to come towards you, because opposites attract, because nature abhors a vacuum, because...do you get it?

It's the opposite, you see. Whatever problem you've got, turn it around and view it by opposite, and you will find the truth of your problem. And once you find the truth of your problem, you will have changed the terminal (the viewpoint of the terminal) and the universe will suddenly change for you...and do the opposite.

So, you're a thief? If you can stop stealing, and I mean in even the smallest, most minute situations, then the universe won't be hiding from you, which is to say, the universe will present itself to you, which is to say, suddenly you will have so much you won't have to steal.

Go on, try it. You'll find it works for one simple reason...you can't argue with the truth.

POSTURE EIGHTY-ONE
Parsva Bakasana (Side Crane Pose)

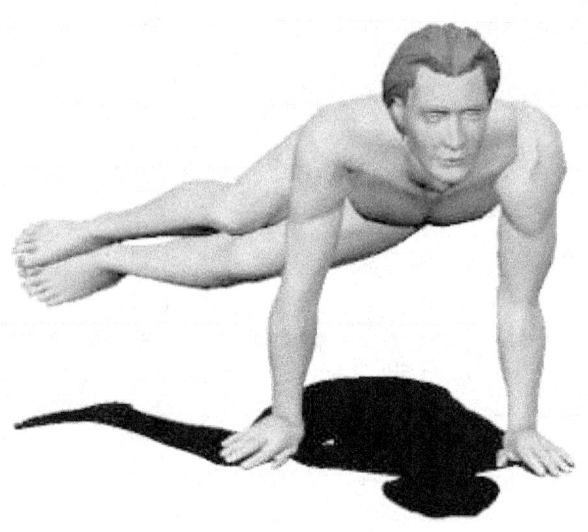

Takes lots of strength, and impeccable balance. Hit a Crane Pose, then simply shift one foot over, put the feet together, and hold the legs to the side, one thigh balanced on the upper arm on the bend just above the elbow.

Relax. Breath. Enjoy.

MORE ON FOR SOMETHING TO BE TRUE....

Continuing the thread of the last discourse...

If you have enemies, then stop being an enemy. Simply, change your viewpoint on one of the terminals of the motor of 'possessing enemies,' and you will suddenly have no enemies. Well, there will still be people who covet your shiny nature, and will want to possess it, but this is simply a case of them still having a motor, and all you have to do is step around the terminal they present and they will be left blundering.

If a person can conquer lust in himself, love from others will replace the void left by that discarded motor.

If a person can stop telling lies, lies will stop being told about him.

If a person can conquer his covetousness, he will suddenly understand the how and why of life.

Do you see how this thing: for something to be true the opposite must also be true, as it pertains to the virtues (and the opposite of virtues) in life?

Look, everything is a motor. Simply grab a terminal, give it a twist of viewpoint, and the motor ceases to function, ceases to have control over you, ceases to be, except as a memory that has no power.

POSTURE EIGHTY-TWO
Tittibhasana (Firefly Pose)

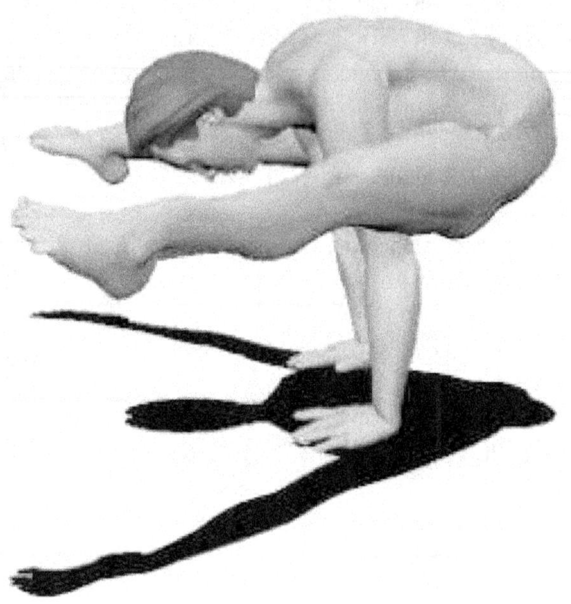

Strong wrists, spread legs, folding at the waist, and concentration...concentration in spades. Do you realize how much pure FOCUS you will have once you can present a pose like the firefly?

Your awareness will be a sharp shard in the eye of darkness, and the world will awake.

Guaranteed. Somewhere on the other side of the planet, the opposite of you will suddenly wake up and say, "Good Lard! Did you feel that? I want to do that, too!"

And, thus, the world awakens to itself as Awareness.

TO BECOME PURE IN ACTION...

To become pure in action is to become pure in thought.
To become pure in thought is to withdraw from the body.
To withdraw from the body is to cease to be a motor for somebody else.
To cease to be a motor for somebody else is to cause them to re-evaluate their life.

"What was that? I was depending on that fellow over in Nigeria to keep my motor in place, to give me cause for existence, to give me a shelf upon which to place my emotions and infatuation with the lives of others. Now that motor is gone, and I am lacking a terminal in the emotions (motions inside the head) that I was depending on to...hmmm. Maybe I could do something else. Something other than hold motors in place that people can get all upset over.

If you do this, if you strike a pose, control yourself, become pure, destroy a motor, then all those that had similar motor, that depended on a belief system of motors to keep existence going on this hellish planet...they lost something in their motor, and...the world awakes.

POSTURE EIGHTY-THREE
Astavakrasana (Eight-Angle Pose)

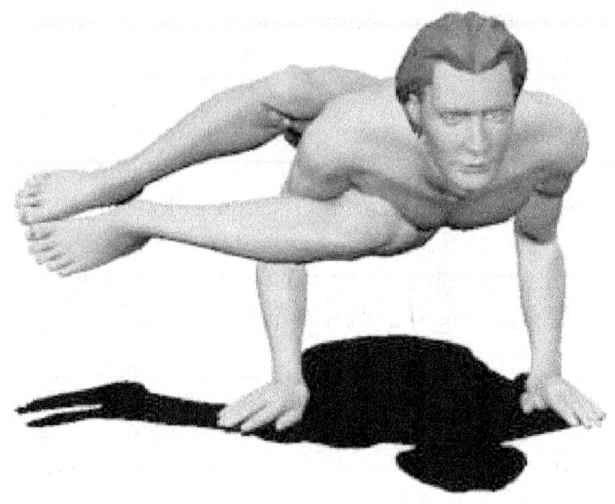

The eight angle pose is similar to the side crane pose. The difference is that you are going to have to work that bottom foot between the arms, then lift it up to place it next to the top foot. Once there you can brace yourself on the body, clamp those legs around the arm and hold on, and it is a pleasure to hold. Be aware, however, that you are going to have to bend the elbows more, and this is going to require different muscles and more strength.

POISE...YOUR ATTITUDE TO LIFE

Poise, how you hold yourself, your attitude towards life, is crucial.

First, it shouldn't take any effort to do the right thing. Simply refuse any breach of morality, or virtue, or any of the principles listed here (see 24 Neutronic Principles), and your life will quickly turn towards the good, and you will encounter a joy you never knew existed as a meat body.

The thing is, you must make a decision to do the right thing, you must set your daily goal as being an embodiment of right action.

To accomplish this decision you must take the principles of right living to heart every day.

Print the basics of a good life towards others on your mirror so that you see it when you shave.

Tape the principles of Neutronics on your door, so that you are reminded to take them into the world outside your door.

At night, take the time to reaffirm your faith in right principles by reading Neutronic Texts and doing Yoga or martial arts.

Even when asleep, you should decide before sleep that you will make a good example of yourself in any dream you might generate or enter.

This is the way to become poised...and to become poised to dive into a life full of riches...a life worth living ten times over!

And, at that point you will be close to not needing an more lives.

POSTURE EIGHTY-FOUR
Mayurasana (Peacock Pose)

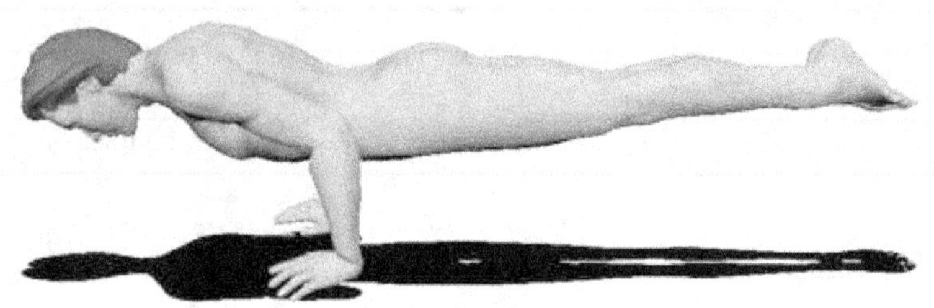

The peacock pose is a close cousin to the four limbed staff pose. All you have to do is shift your weight slightly forward as you lift your legs. Easy squeezy, eh?

Still, if you have been doing your work up to this point, making sure you spent enough time in every posture, even the easy ones, then it should be easy for you.

THE LIFE FORCE

As you close in on Black Belt, and run joyously through these final postures, you may have realized something.

You are (or will be shortly) perceiving life force. This is to say that you have become aware, and you are perceiving awareness.

You cannot see Awareness with the perceptic tools of the body like the eye and the ear and so on. Awareness is invisible to the meat.

But, when one begins to outgrow the need for physical perception tools, and starts discovering his awareness as a way to perceive the world, he also finds that he can see Awareness. He can recognize another person who has achieved realization of awareness, and therefore emits awareness as part of his life.

And, one can see the life force, which is the subtle field (ocean) of awareness upon which this universe rests, and through which we, as aware human beings, swim.

As more and more people become aware of this life force, this ocean of chi, this field of Prana, this stuff of which we are made in truth, then their abilities will manifest.

Healing by laying on the hands. Adjustments of energy fields. Prediction of universal events. All manner of abilities will become the norm for a civilization that has awoken to their true spiritual, aware nature.

POSTURE EIGHTY-FIVE
Urdhva Dhanurasana (Upward Bow or Wheel Pose)

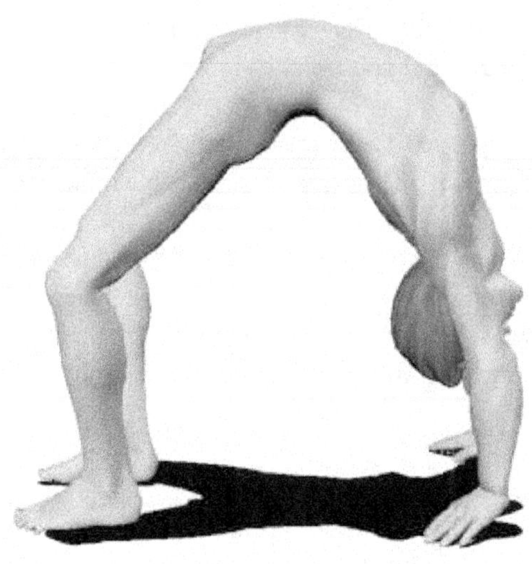

A simple back bend. Anybody can do it, right? Especially if they have just dedicated a year or two to developing complete and total control of their body. Take your time developing this one, and enjoy.

Relax. Breath.

Enjoy.

THE LIGHT OF YOU

An interesting thing: you are a creature of light.

You see, you project the universe, and you do this by manipulating the 'sea of chi,' or prana, or whatever, with your awareness.

Remember, you do not take in light, except in a gross illusion of seeing sunlight.

Rather, you emit the subtle prana energy that generates the universe.

And this prana IS a form of light. Be it subtle and soft and the stuff of you...the soul.

Sometimes, when a person is truly spiritual, full of life, helping to all people, you can see his light. It is like he glows, like his eyes have extra light.

But he is just tapping into the life force, has more life force to give.

And you have managed to see without eyes for a brief moment.

Finishing this course you will begin to emit your own light. You'll probably notice it first in light-hearted laughter, but shortly you will begin to perceive yourself differently, see a glow about your face in the mirror, notice that you are enjoying people oh, so much.

Good.

POSTURE EIGHTY-SIX
Kapotasana (King Pigeon Pose)

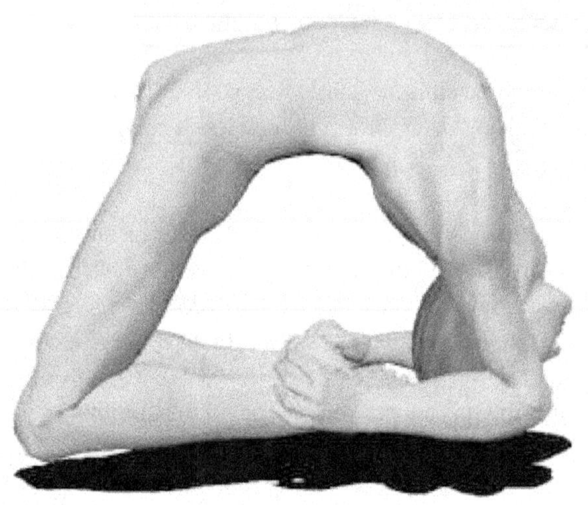

King Pigeon Pose. Very relaxing. Very revealing. You are almost at the end...which is to say, you are almost the beginning of you.

WHAT IT ALL DEPENDS ON

It all depends on you. Everything in the universe. It all depends on your ability to control yourself, to focus yourself as Awareness.

You must give up the meat, be willing to help and share in the glory of existence.

You must be willing to give up motors, put aside distractions, cause yourself to relax, instead of resist.

To put aside your illusive self that your true self may manifest.

The odd thing is that you have been living the truth all your life. You have been in charge of everything...but you have been lying about it.

Silly you.

POSTURE EIGHTY-SEVEN
Urdhva Prasarita Eka Padasana (Standing Split)

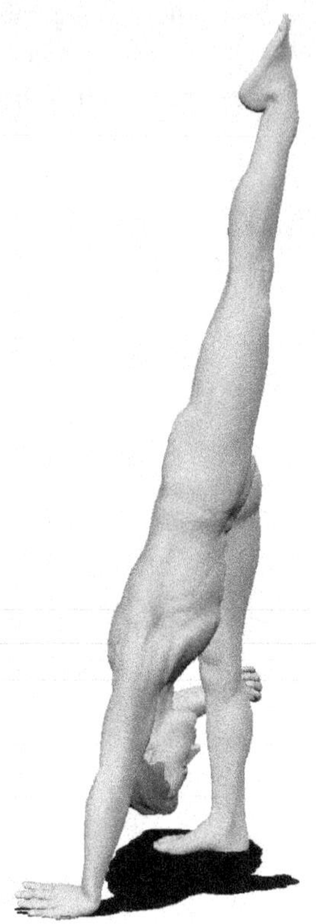

The Standing Splits, a real piece of work.

What's fun is to start with two hands down, then grab the leg with one hand (as shown), and finally grab the leg with both hands, or pray, or something.

Be the first on your block!

THE ULTIMATE CONTROL

Control the body.
Get rid of distractions.
Control emotions.
Get rid of more distractions.
Follow the principles.
Control the mind.
Take control of your motors.
Control yourself.
Learn how to focus the Awareness of yourself.
Learn how to control the light that is you.
Become cognizant of the Greater Awareness of All.

You are back where you started, millions and zillions of lifetimes ago.
And the second bunch of things you have to do starts with one simple command.

Help somebody control their body.

POSTURE EIGHTY-EIGHT
Bhujapidasana (Shoulder-Pressing Pose)

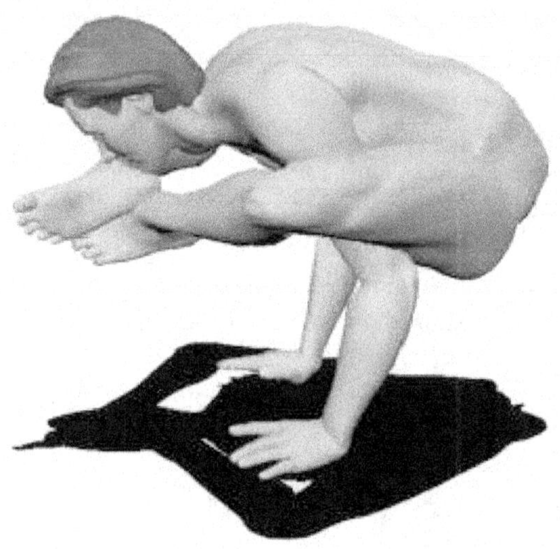

Very good for the shoulders. Lots of power. And, of course, lots of balance. I really enjoy these little arm standers. I remember doing them in PE back when I was in high school a half a century ago.

We did them for kicks and fun games, and they turn out, if you tweak them a bit and learn about meditation, good for the mind and spirit and even Awareness of All.

THE ULTIMATE MEDITATION

Many people have no idea what meditation is. They are given vague instructions, and left to wallow.

Eventually, the form will take hold and guide, but this is a lackadaisical and inefficient way to get anywhere.

It's like tossing somebody a map that has been all balled up and soaked in water so that it will rip if anybody tried to unfold it, and then telling them to read the instructions.

Sheesh.

So let me repeat the definition of meditation you read in the beginning of this epistle.

Attention is fixing your awareness on something.

Meditation is holding your attention (on something) for a prolonged period of time.

Contemplation is holding your attention on something with the intent of perceiving it directly (as it is), and thus ridding yourself of separation from the object (your creation).

When you master meditation, in all its aspects, you achieve the illumination of perception (you become aware that you can be aware of something without the need for eyes, ears, and so on.

The point here is to look out at the universe so intently that you are freed from mental machinations, and realize yourself as Awareness separate from meat.

POSTURE EIGHTY-NINE
Scorpion Variation

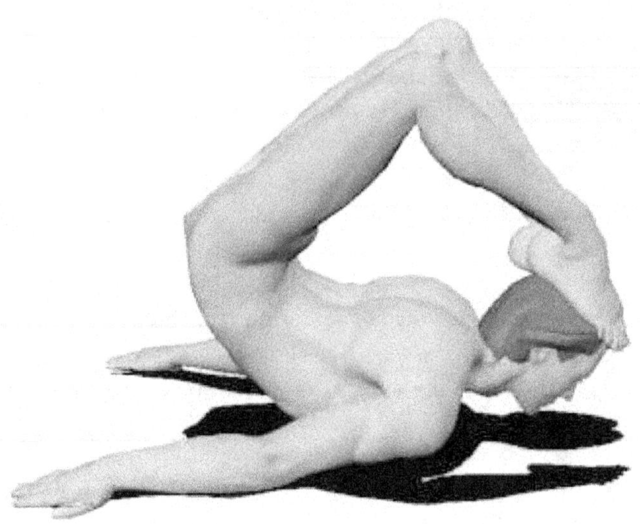

I call this one the Scorpion Variation. I'm sure it has a name, but I am terrible with names. I just care if I can do it...what does it mean...where will it lead me as an Awareness.

The regular scorpion is done on an elbow stand or hand stand, which would turn this 90 degrees on its head.

Great stuff.

ALMOST THERE!

One more pose to do!

Have you started planning for what is next?

I am hoping that you have availed yourself of the Yogata book, and are doing the actual Yogata Kata.

And, I am hoping you have decided to discover martial arts.

Heck, you already have the physical side of it down, and you understand that you exist as an Awareness, so wouldn't it be nice to learn how to use force and flow to manipulate anything in the universe?

Yes, you should continue to do Yoga, and to improve at an accelerated rate. But somebody who gets stuck in one field is not really learning. In the martial arts, past a certain point, you are plumbing your depths, or, as the Japanese say, 'Polishing your soul.'

So you should continue to polish your soul in Yoga, but you should expand your awareness to other fields. Find out how to use Yoga, how to apply it to the positions in the martial arts.

But, it's up to you.

At any rate, thank you for persisting, for coming this far. now, ready for the last pose?

It's a real treat, one of my favorites.

POSTURE NINETY
One Legged Squat Prayer

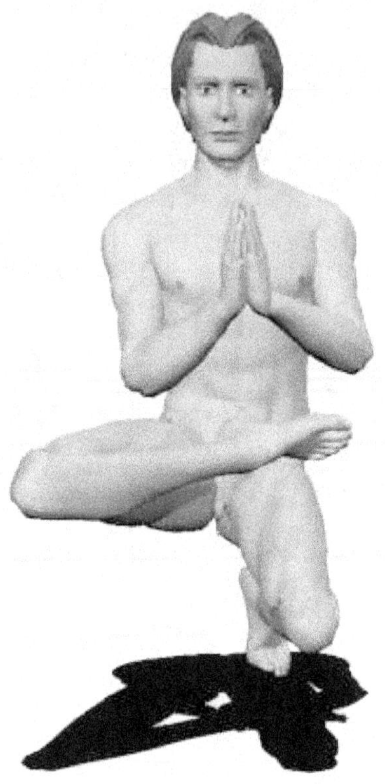

There it is, the one legged Squat Prayer. Deep balance with lots of room for variation.

It's fun to move the arms while trying to stave off the shimmy in the foot and ankle.

So...you know what comes now.

Relax. Breath. Enjoy.

BLACK BELT

Congrats! Big time Congrats!

If you video yourself doing the poses, and the Yoga Kata out of Yogata, I will send you a certificate for Black Belt in yoga. Simply send me the video, or just upload it to a youtube private channel, or whatever other method you prefer for sending videos.

Now, as I asked earlier, what now?

I suggest doing some martial arts. You can take a look at my Martial Arts at MonsterMartialArts.com.

Also, I suggest you delve deeper into Neutronics. I wrote a book on it.

I'll write a couple of pages concerning these suggestions later in the book.

And, I suggest you continue your studies of Yoga. I have included a few illustrations of super advanced studies, and I want you to think about something.

Black Belt means expert. There are, however, rankings beyond black belt. In the martial arts a fourth black belt is a Master. And, in my system of martial arts, there are specific courses to make one an instructor.

So, a lot of roads have opened up to you, and I wish you well, and I trust I will see you down the road.

Thanks, and, again, congrats.

Al Case

YOUR NEXT MEDITATION

I hope you have much benefit in the meditations I have offered in this tome. If you haven't simply do the book again. Heh.

Seriously, while there is still much to be gained from yoga meditation, you will actually progress faster and further, and wake up abilities you never knew you had, if you do the martial arts.

In the martial arts you will learn to...

look into forever better
fix your attention with more power
fix your attention on more detail
create geometries of energy
create space
become more resistant to the ill will of others
find different modes of health which are not available in Yoga
discover potentials of motion you would never find in Yoga
learn how to manipulate the universe through force and flow
refine the mind further
still ever more distractions
become more detailed in your viewpoint of life and living
and so on.

Martial Arts have been called 'The Moving Meditation.'
Unfortunately,
they aren't taught that way much.
But,
in the Matrix Martial Arts courses,
and especially in Neutronics,
you will find that moving meditation.

POSTURE NINETY-ONE
The Holy Crud!
Eka Pada Koundiyanasana II (Pose Dedicated to the Sage Koundinya II)

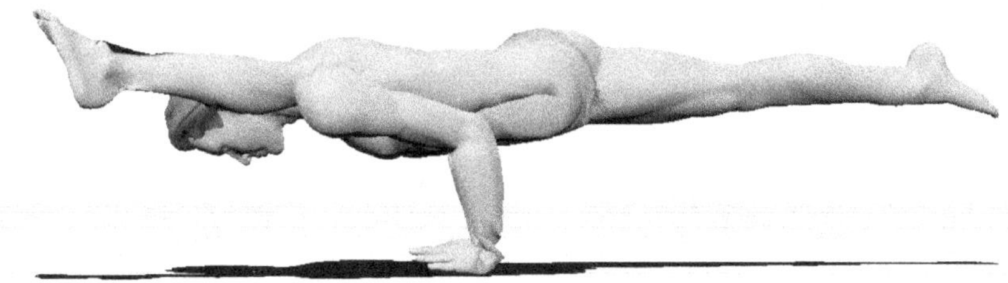

POSTURE NINETY-TWO
The Wachamacallit

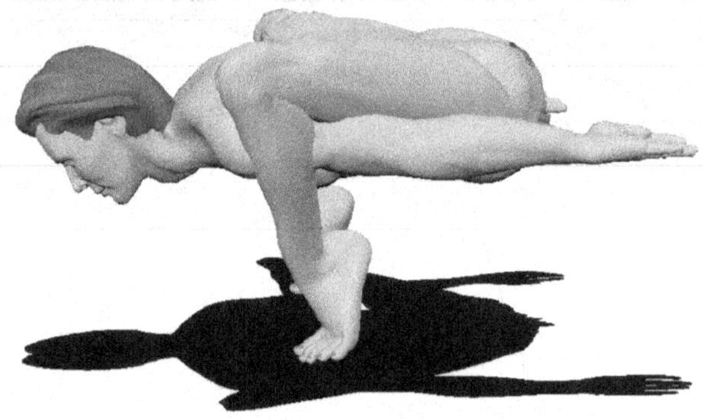

POSTURE NINETY-THREE
The Doodad

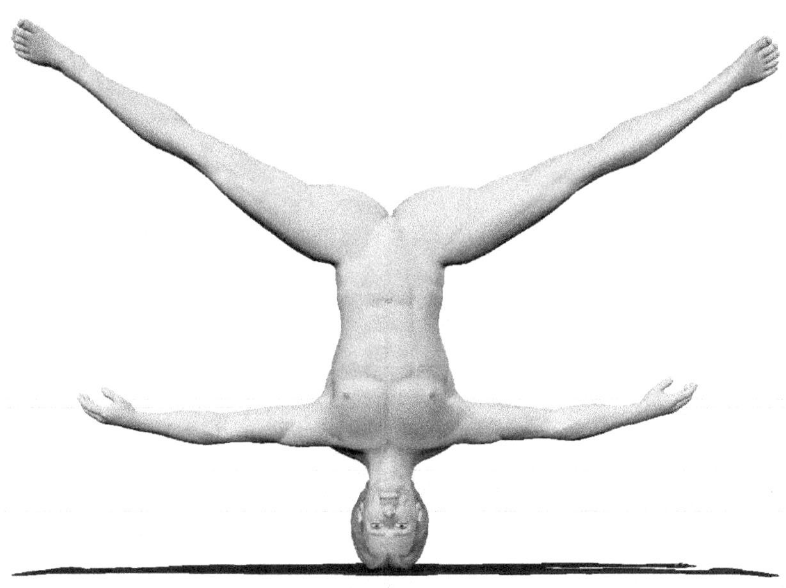

POSTURE NINETY-FOUR
The Doohickey
Pose of the sage Ruchiki (Ruchikasana)

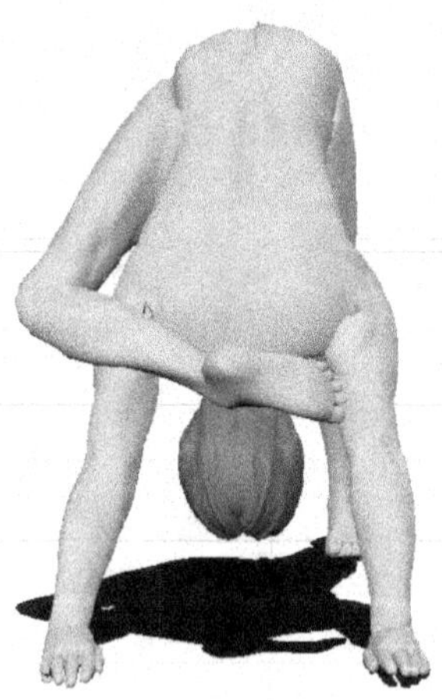

POSTURE NINETY-FIVE
The Goshwally
Pose of the Sage Gheranda (Gherandasana)

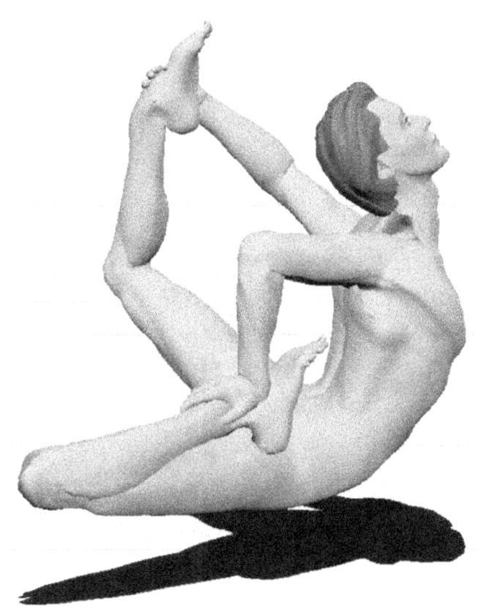

POSTURE NINETY-SIX
The Thingamajig
Formidable Face Pose (Ganda-Bherundasana)

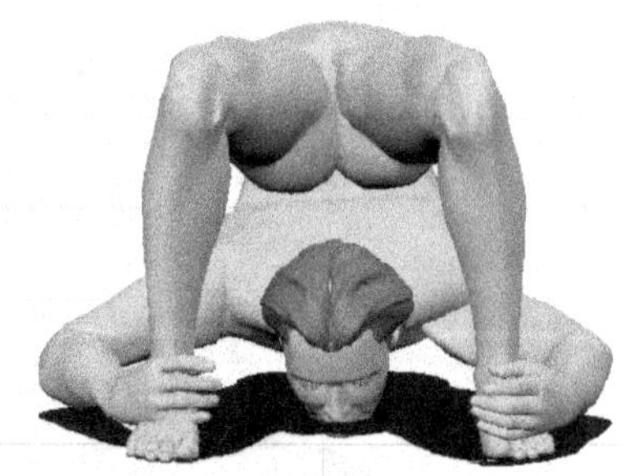

POSTURE NINETY-SEVEN
The Fornsplatt Doodlehopper
Tip Toe Pose (Prapadasana)

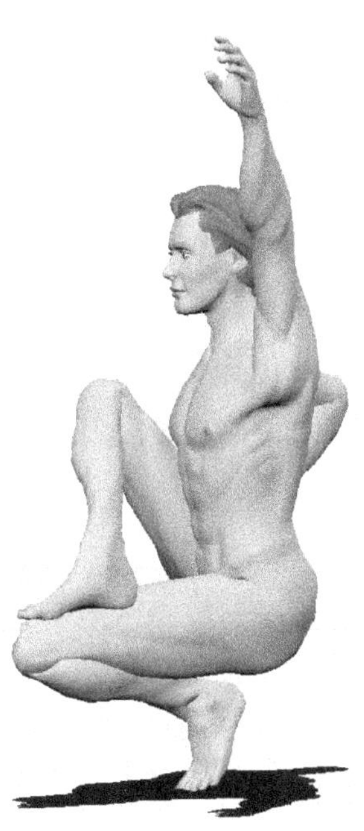

POSTURE NINETY-EIGHT
The Zing Zong Blafadoo
Reclining Angle Pose (Supta-Konasana)

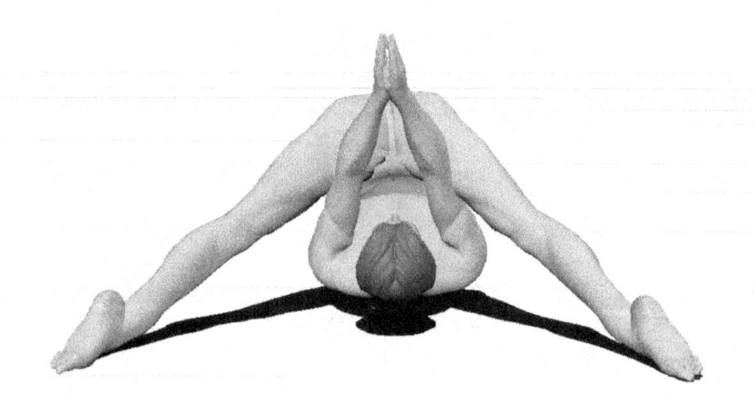

POSTURE NINETY-NINE
The Flacky Wacky Spling Splot
One Hand Lotus Hand Stand (Eka-Hasta-Padma Adho-Mukha-Vrkshasana)

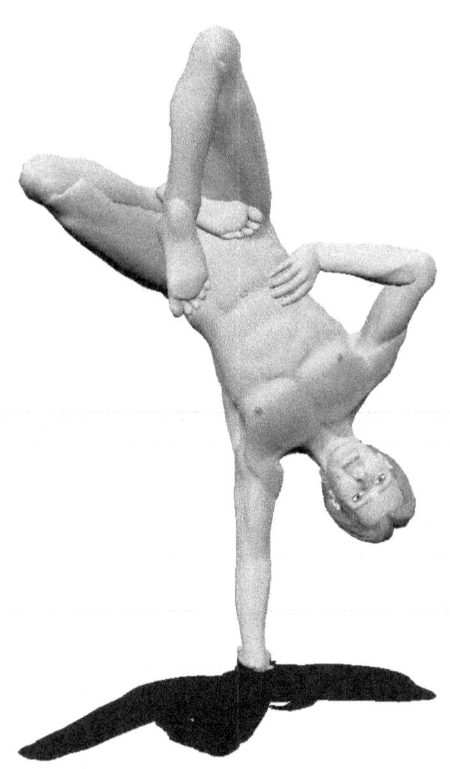

POSTURE ONE HUNDRED
The Don't Touch Anything or I'll Explode Pose

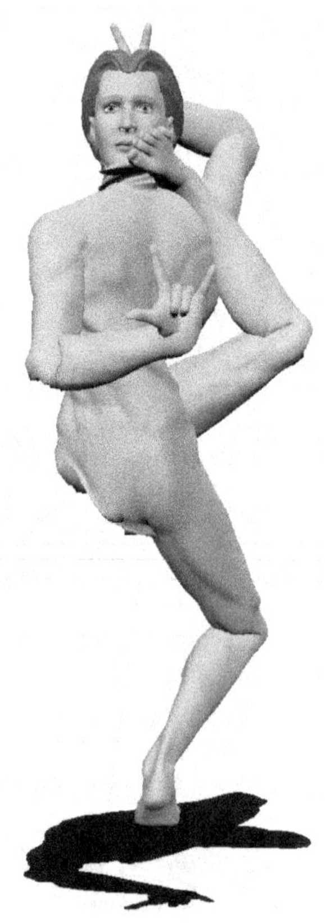

YOGATA
(The Yoga Kata)

The Yoga Kata is probably the best thing to ever happen to Yoga. This is because it opens up the practice of Yoga, and presents a new standard for yogic routines and practice.

When you go to a yoga class you are given a couple of poses, and you work them, spend some time on variations, and the teacher encourages you.

But, the poses are invariably a small cross section of Yoga. 'We are going to work on the hips today.' Or, 'We are going to examine the shoulders this class.'

But what happened to the whole body?

Look, there comes a time when somebody should look at the fine details. But, what you really want, from the get go, is the whole picture. You want to understand how the whole body works, not just one part of it. And you want to understand how the whole body works BEFORE you go looking at the various parts.

Now, you have heard me talk about matrixing, and there have been a few examples, but it is difficult to matrix details before one has the whole picture.

In Yogata (The Yoga Kata), I apply Matrixing to the whole body of Yoga.

It's funny, in the martial arts I always hear people saying, 'Oh, I know what he's doing.' But then they get one of my courses, and their eyes open, and they ALWAYS say, 'OMG! I didn't know he was doing this!'

That's because Matrixing has never been seen; it is a field of knowledge, of logic, really, that has never been seen on planet earth.

In Matrixing you take all the principles of a field, you arrange them in logical order, and you go through combinations, searching for what you don't know.

Not for what you know, which is what everybody looks for, and which is comfortable and same old same old.

But for the uncomfortable knowledge that you didn't know existed.

In the Yogata Kata I matrix the postures to get it all, and I arrange it in the best sequence possible, and the results are magical.

THE FINAL WORD

Thank you.

Al Case

Look for books and courses by Al Case at

MonsterMartialArts.com

AlCaseBooks.com

or on the internet.

www.ingramcontent.com/pod-product-compliance
Lightning Source LLC
Chambersburg PA
CBHW071408150726
48000CB00001B/221